Houses of Sand

Memories of Saudi Arabia

by

Judy MacDonnell

Houses of Sand

Copyright © 2011 by Judy MacDonnell

Cover Art by Laura Shinn

(To view more of Laura Shinn's works or cover designs, visit: www.laurashinn.com)

ISBN-10: 1461111242
ISBN-13: 978-1461111245

This book is licensed for your personal enjoyment only. It may not be copied or reproduced in any manner without express written permission of the author or publisher.

Thank you for respecting the hard work of this author.

Houses of Sand is a personal memoir. Names and other details of the stories herein have been changed to protect the privacy of the individuals concerned.

Cover picture: Escarpment near Riyadh.

DEDICATED TO:
ZALIKHAH

SPECIAL THANKS TO:
Penny, Josie, Susan, Norma, and my husband, who tirelessly edited and advised.

CONTENTS

	Author's Note	vii
1	Welcome to a New World	1
2	The Magic Kingdom	5
3	Beginnings	13
4	Out and About in Al Khobar	33
5	Kidnapped!	41
6	Within the Walls	46
7	Life in the Aramco Lane	53
8	Out in the Sandpit	60
9	Forbidden Love	74
10	Tying the Knot, Shiite Style	77
11	The First King	82
12	Friends and Acquaintances	110
13	Weekend Escape	117
14	Gold, Frankincense and My First Christmas	132
15	First Repat	137
16	In Trouble	148
17	The Biggest Oasis	156

18	Black Pearls	161
19	Playing Trains	169
20	Getting to the Bottom of Things	180
21	Differences	186
22	On being Strung Along	197
23	Tying the Knot, Sunni Style	202
24	Red Sails in the Sunset	206
25	Bad Apples	210
26	Law and Order	214
27	Showcase in the Desert	220
28	A Woman's Place	226
29	Big Hill	232
30	Back in the Sand Pit	246
31	Gated!	256
32	Ravens, Rats and Saudi Arabian Cats	263
33	On the Mat	269
34	A Burning Question	279
35	Hard Pressed	286
36	To Have or to With-hold?	294
37	An Ancient Land	300

38	Black Thursday	306
39	Tying the Knot, Aussie Style	309
40	Casual or Casualty?	314
41	A Slip of the Finger	320
42	The Biggest Sandpit of All	323
43	Oops!	338
44	A Hole in One	345
45	Exit Only	350

Author's Note

I spent the greater part of the 1990s in Saudi Arabia, working for the giant oil company of Saudi Aramco. The boom time of the 1970s and 80s had passed, and lifestyle and company benefit restrictions had affected expatriates in the camps to some extent.

However, the benefits of "Mother Aramco" were still numerous. Repatriation benefits and shipping allowances were generous, and housing was cheap and comfortable. Travel within Kingdom was unimpeded and never did we feel threatened or in danger in any of our desert wanderings. I look back with nostalgia on the wonderful things I was privileged to see and do.

In writing this book I hope to show the personal side of an expatriate's life and work in the Kingdom of Saudi Arabia. It was perhaps the most interesting six and a half years of my life and during this time I gained much respect and admiration for this country and its people.

And so I invite the reader to come with me to a land still unavailable to the casual traveler, to a place where the ancient touches the modern yet retains its charm and dignity, to a land we called the Magic Kingdom.

JUDY MACDONNELL

1- WELCOME TO A NEW WORLD

THE PLANE SLAMMED onto the runway, weaved and bobbed, then slowed to a walking pace. I pressed my face against the window, straining to see through a foggy yellow glow. The Asian flight attendant had bid me a "good fright," when I boarded. Maybe he knew something I didn't. The plane paused as though considering its possibilities before rolling to a stop in front of the terminal building. Finally the doors burst open and passengers began to spew out onto the steaming tarmac.

Soon it was my turn to grab hand luggage and stumble down the steps. It was only two in the morning, but humidity engulfed me in its clammy arms. The area was lit up like a Hollywood stage, the lights joining forces with the weather to start rivulets of perspiration flowing within the dark and modest outfit I'd worn for my entry into this Muslim country. I was the antithesis of a movie star.

Like an immense and drunken millipede, the line of passengers wobbled into the airport terminal. A blast of cold air stung my wet skin as I entered the building. I was the only female in the line that settled in front of the customs desk under Foreign Passports. All of the other passengers were men—from places like India, Pakistan, Sri Lanka and the Philippines, seeking, I guessed, a fast buck in the land I came to know as the Magic Kingdom. Everyone stood quietly and only the clang of luggage carts echoed in the great hall.

"Can I hook up with you going through customs? It's quicker if they think you're a couple."

I spun around, startled at the English accent. A gloomy white face peered into mine.

"Sure, where are you going?" I asked.

"The British Aerospace compound in Dammam. I've just been out on leave. What about you?"

I shrugged. "Don't know, really. I'm starting work with Aramco as a Physical Therapist. I think someone is supposed to meet me here."

"Aramco, eh. Lucky you; it's very comfortable on their compounds. Americans really know how to look after themselves. Most of these guys here are contractors, coming to work for a few dollars a day for various companies. Poor buggers won't get to go home again for several years."

I glanced again at the gaunt brown figures ahead and felt guilty at my good fortune.

"Crazy place, this," said the Englishman. "You'll get to know the ropes after a while. Doesn't take long. Hot as hell and some idiotic customs, but the pay is good."

"It's hot all right," I said. "It's eighty-five degrees at two in the morning!"

Someone left the customs desk and everyone else moved forward one pace. My self-appointed companion kicked his carry-on bag along the floor behind me.

"It's going to get worse," he said. "It's only May. And what kind of country is it where the men dress themselves in white and keep their women in stinking-hot black?"

"It feels like a different planet here. I didn't see much coming in except a lot of lights."

"They always bring you in at night," he said sagely. "Because if you could see what the place was really like, you'd turn around and go straight back home."

Suddenly an official in a white robe appeared at the head of the line, his eyes searching. He flicked the ends of his white headscarf up over his head then beckoned in my direction. I panicked—did he want me? What had I done? I had barely arrived; was I in trouble?

"You'd better go," said the Englishman with a sigh. "There goes my quick trip through customs. You're a female—they want you out of here."

I plucked myself from the line and stepped toward the little man in white.

"Come!" he said, ushering me through immigration with a smile and a nod. I handed over my passport to the immigration officer, remembering not to look him in the eye. The recruiting officer back in Australia has said it could be misconstrued as a come-on.

A tall, slender Arab, hand outstretched, stepped forward and exchanged greetings in Arabic with my guide. Then he nodded to me.

"Hello! My name is Salim," he said in impeccable English. "Did you have a good flight?"

I shook his hand, grateful to find the common ground of hospitality between the distant familiarity of home and this strange new country I was entering.

I'd brought only one suitcase and, as soon as I collected it from the carousel, an Indian porter attached himself to it. He stuck to it like a leech until we'd left customs and reached the exit doors. Then I realized I had no riyals with which to pay him. There was only a UK ten pound note in my purse.

"That is OK," said the porter, his eyes glinting. I shook my head.

Salim thrust a ten riyal note at the porter. He took it and faded away, and Salim led me outside to a white van. I fell into air conditioning and a heavenly-soft red velvet seat, and suddenly my tension drained away. Being a woman in Saudi Arabia was not going to be all bad!

2 - THE MAGIC KINGDOM

BRRRRRINGGGG! MY EYES flew open in a panic—oh! It was only the alarm clock. I allowed a minute for my heart to slow down. Then I rubbed the grit from my eyes, rolled out of bed with all the enthusiasm of a rock, and landed with a thud on the floor. I'd had precisely three hours of sleep.

The taxi had arrived in the main Aramco compound of Dhahran at about three-thirty in the morning. After much fruitless searching for the key to my new apartment, Salim had decided to drop me off at the company's guest accommodations for the rest of the night.

"I'll come and get you at eight-thirty in the morning," he'd promised. "And I will have the key to your apartment. We'll go shopping." I'd set the alarm for seven-thirty.

I washed my face in the bathroom and tried to make the best of my bleary blue-eyed countenance. My streaky brown-and-blonde hair insisted on waving the wrong way. I thought my clothing was fairly acceptable, considering the lack of an iron, and hung not too badly over my slender (let's face it—*skinny*) body. At thirty-six I still looked fairly youthful, but this morning's lack of sleep was a definite disadvantage to my appearance.

I ate some cereal from a food parcel in the kitchen, which looked through an arched opening into a combined lounge and dining area. Through the window I saw nothing but sand. In the bathroom were the toilet, hand basin and a bathtub with a shower and curtain. The bedroom was large, with a double bed under the window. There was a blank wall opposite this window.

After dressing, I dared to explore my immediate territory. Beyond the entry door the halls in the apartment building were empty, the doors to other apartments locked. I wondered what lay beyond the main doors of the building but dared not wander too far in case Salim called while I was away.

Salim didn't show at eight-thirty. Time passed. Ten o'clock. Then eleven o'clock. Questions boiled in my mind. *What kind of a place had I come to? And where was Salim?* The panic and uncertainty of the previous night struck again.

Why was I here, anyway? Why hadn't I stayed in Australia within my comfort zone? My family was used to moving about. They'd both been school teachers with a desire to help educate those in less fortunate countries than their own. I'd grown up in such remote places as the Cook Islands and Samoa, in the days when regular flights were unheard of and books and groceries came in on a six-monthly supply ship.

My otherwise supportive parents had become increasingly concerned as I'd read to them news items I'd gleaned from books and magazines about Saudi Arabia. Just two days previously my father had said, "The more I hear about this place the less I like the idea of you going there." Their faces had been a picture of concern as they'd waved goodbye at the airport in Sydney.

Several months previously I'd realized that I was making little headway against the bills accrued since building a small house. At this point, I'd had the bright idea of applying to work for Saudi Aramco, the largest oil company in the world, which was based in the eastern province of Saudi Arabia.

"Please send your résumé in immediately," the agent had said on the phone. "Someone is interviewing for Aramco Medical next week."

The interviewer was Abdalla, the supervisor of Rehabilitation in the company. He had gone through my résumé point by point. It was almost like a test, I mused, to see if I'd remembered what I'd written down.

He wound up by asking if I'd ever married, and when I said no, he wondered how I had 'escaped'—at the ripe old age of thirty-six. Then he asked me how long I planned to stay in Aramco, should I get the job. I suggested I might go for a year.

He shook his head sadly.

"I am interviewing you for a special job, to set up a new physical therapy unit in a clinic away from the main compound. We would want someone for two years or more for this job. What would entice you to stay longer?"

I thought for a moment. Even if they offered me a good wage, I wouldn't stay if I was unhappy.

"If I like the work and the people I work with, I would stay longer," I said finally.

The next day a phone call assured me that I had the job. But it was to be five months before all the preliminaries were over and I could start work. The lists went on and on. Complete dental x-rays, a full medical examination, audiology tests, references from all previous employment, notarized copies of all documents... And Aramco paid for all of it, even the transportation, asking only for the receipts so they could reimburse me.

Even after these evidences of Aramco's care and consideration, I felt very vulnerable and uncertain. Mustering all the obstinacy of my Scottish and German ancestry, I determined not to give in to my fears. There must be a phone book somewhere around—and there it was, in a drawer below the phone. All the company departments were listed. *Which one to call?* Personnel?

After half a dozen calls I got lucky. Yes, the secretary knew Salim. Yes, he was the same Salim who had picked me up the previous night. He should have come to collect me by now; she'd call his home and get back to me.

A few minutes later the phone rang—Salim's wife had informed the secretary that he was still asleep in bed. He'd be in after lunch. I sighed with relief and stretched out on the knobbled white sofa to read through my orientation notes for the twentieth time.

Salim arrived at five thirty. He smiled as I opened the door to his knock.

"Would you like to go shopping now?"

"Don't you think the shops will be closed?" I asked.

"Maybe," he replied doubtfully. "Anyway, here is the key to your new apartment. Are you ready to come?"

"Ummm, I think so."

My new apartment was identical to the one I had been in all day, but was on the ground floor of a residential block bustling with life. Apartments sprouted on both sides of a long corridor that ran the length of the building; the layout was the same for the two floors above, apart from a laundry on the middle floor.

My apartment opened out through a sliding glass door onto a little outdoor patio where dry sticks, propped against a high concrete wall, proved that there had once been a garden.

I found bed linens, kitchen utensils, saucepans, cutlery and dishes in the cupboards—everything one could possibly need. A large package of groceries in the kitchen would nourish me until I could get to the grocery store and stock up. Gratitude to my new employer surged within me. And then exhaustion took over and I fell into bed.

The next morning I reported for orientation. My guide, Martha, was a friendly American woman with Big Hair and impeccable makeup. She explained the workings of the company before driving me around the compound of Dhahran.

Aramco was huge. It used more paper than any other organization in the world, apart from the White House, and provided all that an employee might need in the way of free medical care, transport, house maintenance, power and water. I would be paid to leave the country every year on repatriation, or 'repat', and a very generous shipping allowance would be mine should I wish to bring anything into Kingdom.

Houses were of many types and sizes, some in rows, others detached. Tall palms lined wide streets; flower gardens bloomed everywhere. It was an oasis in the desert. Martha pointed out the school, the swimming pool and other recreational facilities, the various mosques on the compound, the administrative hub surrounded by fences, the oil wells on the perimeter. There was almost reverence in the way she spoke of the well called simply 'Dammam number seven,' the first well to have produced oil in four years of fruitless searching.

At the post office in the Al Mujammah building, I was given a mailbox and a code to open it and then we moved on to the grocery store, commonly known as the commissary.

"Most items you might need are stocked here," said Martha. "Of course, it always pays to check that you have all your ingredients before starting a recipe, in case the commissary doesn't have something. You may find that they've run out of chocolate chips, for example, or waffles, and won't have any more for a few months. When something comes in, people often buy up and hoard it in case they don't see it again for a while!"

I thought back to my childhood on a remote island in the South Pacific, where we had lived mainly on local produce supplemented with bins of weevilly flour and powdered milk, and where shipments only arrived at six-monthly intervals. Life would not, I decided, be too difficult without chocolate chips or waffles.

Everything depended on the oil industry. When oil prices rode high, the company did too. Recruiting increased, new buildings went up, services expanded. When the oil industry took a dive, the company tightened its belt. Employees were offered retirement packages; buildings and occasionally entire compounds, were 'mothballed,' locked up to bake in the sun until they were required again.

Several Aramco compounds had been built around the Arabic peninsula. Some were family compounds but others, particularly in remote areas, were for working men only. I, as a female, would be working, of course, in a family compound.

After a thorough tour of Dhahran and a buffet lunch at a five star hotel near the airport, my head was spinning. When I was finally dropped off in the late afternoon near my apartment building, three young women approached.

"Are you Judy?" one of them said hesitantly.

"Yes," I replied, mystified.

With squeals of delight they introduced themselves—my new co-workers! Maria, a bouncy American with sparkling blue eyes would be my immediate boss. Smooth-skinned, tanned Jeannie was a New Zealander and Seaghdha was an Irish lass with a head of black curls.

They all spoke at once and I was overwhelmed. I had never felt more welcomed in my life.

"You'll be here for a month or so before you start work in RT," Maria said.

I stared at her, not understanding.

"Oh my goodness," she whispered, glancing guiltily at the others, "you haven't been told yet, have you!"

What?" I asked frantically. The blood in my veins felt cold.

"I'm so sorry—you should have been told earlier. You won't be staying here in Dhahran with us. You're going to be working in Ras Tanura," she said. "Starting a new physical therapy clinic."

I leaned against a wall, stunned, and suddenly remembered what the interviewer had said several months ago—I was needed to start a new physical therapy unit away from the main compound. My new friends suddenly seemed to fade out of reach.

And then a picture came to mind of a white beach and blue water, which I had seen during my orientation in far away Australia. A picture taken at the place called Ras Tanura, which seemed more like a seaside resort than a company compound. My pulse began to quicken.

3 - BEGINNINGS

"MY FIANCÉ AND I are going out to eat in Khobar tonight," Maria said. "Would you like to come with us? Dean and I could pick you up in an hour or so."

I was suffering from jetlag and my head felt as if it was beginning to float away from my body, but it seemed a pity to pass up this opportunity.

"Thanks, I'd love to," I said.

"Khobar is the nearest town to us," said Maria. "It costs ten riyals, about three dollars, to get a taxi but Dean usually drives me in."

I liked Dean immediately. He was quite a bit taller than Maria and well-built, with an open, friendly face. They were a handsome couple. We drove through the gates of the compound and were speeding along a modern four-lane highway when a sudden thought struck me.

"Oh no!"

"What's the matter?" cried Maria.

"I just realized—we're in this vehicle together and none of us are married! Won't we get into trouble?"

Maria and Dean rocked with laughter.

"That's the case in some parts of Arabia," Maria said, "but here in the Eastern Province we have more freedom. Nobody has ever challenged us and we travel together all the time. "

"If ever you are walking with a man and a religious policeman, a *mutawa*, approaches though, the man should walk off and pretend he doesn't know you," Dean piped up. "A woman is safer on her own than with a man."

"Really?" I asked. "Why is that?"

"Because *mutawas* are not allowed to touch women, or even to speak with them, actually. A man can be dragged away to jail, but if a woman is doing something wrong, they can't touch her. If she is with a man, the man is automatically to blame for not controlling her."

Maria told me of a couple who had been stopped by a *mutawa* in Riyadh. A man had offered to drive his friend's wife to town as his friend couldn't take her. The mutawa asked them if they were married and they said, "Yes." After examining their papers carefully he said, "You may both be married, but not to each other!"

There was so much to learn. I felt so comfortable with these two. They were just like family.

"Call me if you need help, anytime," said Dean. "We guys are aware of the difficulties women have in getting around here. You can't drive. We can, and we're happy to help you out."

"What about clothing?" I asked. "I understand that we don't have to wear the *abaya*, or black cloak, that the Arabian women wear."

"Right," said Maria. "In some areas of Saudi Arabia the expat women have to wear *abayas* and sometimes even headscarves, but here we only have to dress modestly. Always have your knees and elbows covered. Long baggy pants are good, and make sure your top is loose and long and you won't get into trouble."

Now the road was fringed with tall palms.

"This is beautiful downtown Khobar," said Dean wryly. "Actually it's a pretty good place to shop. You can find just about anything you want here if you know where to look."

Squat, flat-roofed concrete buildings lined the streets, and litter over steps and sidewalks of varying levels lent a shabby touch to the scene. On either side of us vehicles jostled, honking horns, revving engines, passing across double lines.

"Defensive driving is part of life here," said Maria. "I don't care at all that females are not allowed to drive, I don't *want* to."

People hurried here and there, some obviously expatriates, but most of them Arabs in traditional dress. Men glided along in flowing white robes (*thowbs*) and white, or red and white checked, head scarves (*guthras*) on their heads. The women, however, were draped from head to toe in black, their faces completely covered.

"How can they see?" I exclaimed.

"They can't." Maria glanced at me sideways. "Not very well anyway, especially when the light isn't good. You'll see Bedouin women with eye slits in their veils, but the town women usually have their eyes covered along with everything else."

I remembered a photo I had seen, at my Aramco orientation in Australia, of a woman smoking a cigarette through the black cloth that covered her face.

"That's the Al Shula Mall," said Dean, pointing out a four storey concrete building, which filled a whole block. "It's a bit down at heels but is the best-known landmark in Khobar. It has gold souks, electronic stores, clothing, food, stationery...anything you can imagine. On the top floor is the Big Apple, a shop that sells great cards and mementoes of Saudi Arabia."

Dean parked on a side street in front of the restaurant.

"Here we are," he said. Through large windows I could see men sitting at small tables. "We'll go upstairs to the family area."

"Females aren't allowed to sit and eat in public," Maria explained. "Single women or families are given special cubicles in restaurants. And actually, it's rather nice to have the privacy."

Our cubicle was shrouded by screens. The Indian waiter brought large jugs of water and Saudi champagne—apple juice mixed with Perrier water. I hadn't realized how thirsty I was.

"We should drink a lot in this heat," Maria said. "It's very easy to become dehydrated."

After the meal, we sat and talked for a short while before Dean and Maria decided it was time to leave. With a seven o'clock start in the mornings, most Aramcons hit the sack early. My head was throbbing by the time we returned to the Dhahran camp.

The next morning I dressed in the uniform I had brought with me from Australia and found my way to the hospital before seven. It was a large, modern building, air-conditioned and bustling with activity.

"Parents must not accompany children when entering the hospital," read signs at the entrance. Yes, English is a strange language, I thought.

Down a flight of stairs from the ground floor, I found the Rehabilitation Unit. There Maria introduced me to James, the Rehabilitation Supervisor. He was tall and thin, with a mass of fair hair and a wide crooked smile.

"Welcome to Saudi Aramco!" he said.

After a tour around the building we returned to his office.

"You'll be in Dhahran for a month, learning the Aramco system and taking some Arabic classes," he said. "And after you start work in Ras Tanura you'll come down for meetings once a week.

"The clinic building in Ras Tanura was built several years ago. It was originally meant to be a hospital with full services. Shortly after it was finished oil prices took a dive and so it was 'mothballed,' never opened as a hospital but gradually, over the years, day clinics were opened.

"We've been planning to open a Physical Therapy Unit there for some time. Now, whenever anyone needs treatment, they have to take a bus down from RT to Dhahran, have their treatment, then catch another bus back. Altogether it takes a minimum of three hours off work. More if the patient misses a bus on either end of the run and has to wait. With you up there, patients will be able to have their treatments and get straight back to work."

"Will I live in Dhahran or Ras Tanura?" I asked.

"Well, you'll have to be in Dhahran for a while, because we don't actually have the equipment for Ras Tanura yet!" he said sheepishly. "It has been ordered and we know it's coming. When the equipment arrives we'll get you started up there. One of our Physical Therapy assistants will go with you for a few weeks until you feel comfortable on your own."

I could hardly wait to visit Ras Tanura and James drove me there a few days later. We sat in air-conditioned comfort in a company car, gazing out through a white-hot haze. A four-lane highway stretched ahead like a black and white striped snake toward the horizon, the sandy plains on either side dotted with scrubby brush and over everything the vivid blue canopy of the sky.

"We don't have a budget," James told me. "If you find you need anything in your work up here, just let me know and I can order it. It will take time to arrive, but it will come."

I marveled at the difference between Aramco and every other place I had ever worked, where space and money for equipment had always been at a premium.

"Look! That's *Qatif*, a Shiite area. It's an oasis." James pointed at trees and grass in the distance, contrasting starkly with the desert through the shimmering haze. "Shiites are a minority sect of Islam here. They are usually the last to get running water, telephones, power…they are at the bottom of the list for employment and are desperate for jobs. A couple of years ago there was a riot, and some of the locals burned a bus. Army troops were sent in and started shooting. Twenty or so Shiites were killed before it was all over. There's some ill-feeling between the Shiites and Sunnis, even now."

We were back to the sandy landscape, and suddenly a ship appeared in the middle of the road. I laughed in surprise.

"That's the Suwani family monument." James chuckled. "The Arabs love big centerpieces as features on their roads and highways. You'll see a lot of it. There's a spaceship in the middle of an intersection in Dammam."

"Interesting!" I said. "In Australia we do the same. We build big pineapples, bananas, mangoes, prawns, sheep, and various other things to catch people's attention."

"Here we are," said James as we rounded a corner. The walls of a large compound stretched before us, palms peeping over them. "Ras Tanura is about three miles long and half a mile wide and lies along the beach front. Everyone in Dhahran rehab unit is jealous of you. I would love to work up here and so would half of Dhahran."

"Why don't you appoint someone else to come here, since it's a solo position?" I wanted to know.

"Wouldn't it make sense to send someone with more Aramco experience here and keep me in Dhahran?"

James shook his head.

"It might make sense to you but it isn't how the company works," he said. "You can't get transferred that easily. You have been recruited for this specific purpose, and so this is where you go."

We flashed our ID cards to the security guard and drove slowly through the gates.

Ras Tanura was a family compound on a peninsula surrounded by the Arabian Gulf. The largest oil refinery in the world smoked silently off one end while the Yacht Club and Hobby Farm (horse stables) sprawled off the other. The community was bordered on three sides by substantial security walls which were punctuated by several gates around its perimeter. Security guards manned each gate to ensure that only those with Aramco ID or those signed in by residents could enter.

It's more like a holiday resort than a residential compound, I mused, as we cruised around the streets. Palms waved, Japanese grass flourished along the roadsides and median strips, and flowers bubbled out of manicured beds. Unlike Dhahran, the streets were almost deserted. They bore names like Beach, Surf, Sandpiper, Sunrise and Egret.

"There's the commissary, or grocery store, where you'll buy your provisions," said James, pointing to large square buildings at the edge of the compound. "There is the mail center, also the hairdresser and community services. You'll have a post box with an access code, as we do in Dhahran."

We coasted past a bus stop where a green and white Mercedes bus was pulling away.

"Buses go between here and Dhahran every hour, even if there is only one person aboard. Transport is free; just show your ID card. So are local telephone calls, all your house maintenance, power and water. You also have free access to the swimming pools, squash and tennis courts, golf course, gymnasium and library."

"Is there anything you have to pay for?" I asked.

"You have to rent your house of course, although it isn't much, and there are small membership fees for any clubs or special groups you choose to join while you're here. There are special groups for photography, computers, sailing, darts, dancing, sports of various kinds, painting, various crafts, and the Arabian Natural History Association. The DOG group, or the Dhahran Outing Group, runs trips to many parts of the world."

"It sounds as though there may not be enough time for work!" I laughed.

We turned around at the sign, "No photography allowed." I knew that the Arabs were justifiably sensitive about security around the refinery. During the Gulf War in 1991 it would have been a prime target for the Iraqis and it was thought that the early strikes from the allies had fortuitously taken out some long-range missiles, which were doubtless aimed at this area.

"Now for the clinic," said James.

We drove down a side street and parked in front of a large, freestanding building with glass doors. As the car door opened, I was greeted by a blast of fiery air. I winced. Air conditioning was not an option in this country—it was a necessity.

Inside the clinic our first stop was to introduce me to the Chief Physician, Dr Bato. He shook my hand warmly.

"We are so pleased you are here," he said. "We've all been waiting for you!"

The Physical Therapy unit was to be in the middle of the building on the ground floor. I was disappointed that there were no windows, but otherwise it was well suited to our purpose. Right now though, the large room was nothing but an empty shell.

"You can have cubicles set up here, here and here," said James. "The parallel bars could be over there against the wall, and that area could be the treatment room. We can put storage shelves in that space and the reception area will be here." He sounded as excited as I felt.

"I think I'm going to enjoy working here," I told him.

"You will have a grade code of ten, the same as a regular therapist in Dhahran, but we'll apply for a grade code of eleven after you get started," said James. "Now, let me show you where you'll be living."

He picked up a key from Personnel, in a long administration building, and drove me to a row of apartments.

"They're called 'windmills' because of their shape on the building plan. In each block are four apartments, which have their own courtyards and storage sheds.

"They are old buildings and will probably soon be replaced, but lots of single employees like them. Of course it is only temporary housing—you'll soon be eligible to bid for permanent housing, if you want to."

Maria had explained the system. Every month a few houses were made available, some for males and some for females, and bids were considered on the basis of time served in the company plus the grade code of the employee. Even with a grade code of ten I would have an advantage over many of the other women on camp, except the female doctors and those who had gained points from long service with the company.

My windmill was small and old, but comfortable. The front door opened into a roomy lounge with a kitchen on one side and a bedroom and bathroom on the other. Guests would have to walk through the bedroom to get to the bathroom, but I could use a screen to advantage. Yes, for the present the windmill would do very nicely indeed. I would look through the Aramco furniture catalogue later to select the furniture I needed.

"OK," said James. "Let's carry on."

He pulled up outside a large building and we got out of the car. I gasped. A band of white, silky sand divided green lawns and palms from the turquoise waters of the Arabian Gulf. Gentle surf rustled over the sand. The shoreline stretched out as far as I could see in both directions with thatch-shaded picnic tables dotting the beach. It was the picture I had seen at orientation in Australia. Salt air tingled in my nostrils. People paid big money to vacation in places like this!

James was watching my reaction, a grin widening across his face.

"I told you, you're the envy of everyone in the Dhahran clinic. Now, let's have lunch."

The Surf House, a community building containing a cafeteria, library, bowling alley, pool hall, various convention rooms and an open area under cover, looked out over the beach. We served ourselves and paid the cashier at the end of the line. It was cafeteria food, but not bad at all. The prices were minimal due to company subsidies.

We returned reluctantly to Dhahran. For a month I reported to work in the Dhahran clinic rehab unit, learning the 'Aramco system.' Malouf, the Lebanese Arabic instructor, worked with me on all the questions and responses I would need to know in Arabic for evaluations and treatments. I attended classes but also had individual lessons, teaching muscles in my mouth and throat to produce sounds I had never imagined possible. I had always enjoyed French lessons at high school and now I found Arabic equally as satisfying.

The computer was one of my greatest concerns. I'd never even laid hands on one before, and was quite afraid of it. Maria carefully wrote out all the instructions I would need to keep statistics for the new unit. She was a kind and gentle guide and was becoming a dear friend.

A computer had been ordered for my new job but would not be forthcoming for some time, so I'd have to do the paperwork twice every day. First in longhand on printed sheets and then, after work, all the information from the day would have to be transferred onto the central system via a computer somewhere else in the clinic.

Aramco ran by computer. Every morning before the workday began, the computers spewed out updated schedules for the appointment desk—in duplicate. The piles of paper were several inches thick. Duplicate pages were automatically discarded or used for scrap.

"I know, it seems wasteful," Maria murmured, "but we don't have single paper sheets and we don't yet have a means of recycling."

When the new equipment arrived, James drove me to Ras Tanura again. He was like a kid on Christmas morning, tearing boxes open, figuring out how to put machines and trolleys together and planning where everything should go.

"I shouldn't be organizing this," he said suddenly, with a laugh. "You're the one who's going to be working here!"

"You're doing a great job," I told him. "I'm grateful for your help."

He chuckled self-consciously when the treatment couches were unwrapped.

"I ordered pink," he said, "because you are a girl."

It was touching that he had taken time out from his administrative work to help with this. His support continued over the next months while I wrestled with the new job, language and culture, although Maria was the one I turned to for help on a day-to-day basis.

On the telephone, I told my parents how thrilled I was with my new job and the many benefits of the company, and they sounded greatly relieved.

"You may as well stay as long as possible and earn as much as you can!" my father said happily.

I moved into my windmill and became permanent in Ras Tanura, but once a week for several weeks I went to Dhahran for Arabic lessons and to talk over problems with James.

One day in Dhahran I wandered into the Al Mujammah building, which housed the mail center amongst other services, to escape the heat. A tall, dark-haired girl passed by and I yelped in recognition. She turned and paused, and we stared at each other.

It seemed a lifetime since we'd met at the Aramco orientation back in Australia. Tanya was one of four secretaries, recruited at the same time as I and who had arrived a month previously. Tanya and Marcia were settled in a large house on the Dhahran campus, Kathy and Monika in Ras Tanura, she told me.

We exchanged phone numbers and vowed to keep in touch. She was working for Security, a job that suited her as she'd had experience in police work before coming to Arabia.

"Something really big is happening and I am busting to tell you about it! But I can't," she would sometimes say.

She never did break the trust of her department, and I was glad she could keep a secret for she had some of mine to keep as time went on.

"You should get in touch with Kathy and Monika," Tanya said. "They really like it in Ras Tanura."

Monika was already involved with a boyfriend and had little time to socialize, but Kathy and I quickly bonded. I loved her warm, confiding nature and whimsical Australian humor. It was refreshing to meet her after work whenever time permitted. Kathy's friends soon became my friends and we shared many evenings of music, good food and laughter.

Ras Tanura welcomed me with open arms. Soon, wherever I walked, people waved or honked their horns as they passed me on the street. And true to his word, Dean was ready to help with transport and helped me choose and bring home a bicycle from Rahima.

This little down-at-heels village sprawled just across the highway from Ras Tanura and owed its existence to the oil company. A hodge-podge of old and new buildings crowded the narrow streets and if you knew where to look you could find anything you needed there. Some of the expatriates on camp didn't venture past it. Actually, some of the expatriates didn't venture anywhere, except to the airport.

Inside the wide doors of the Singer Store, fabrics from Europe and the United States jostled alongside craft supplies, Indian knick-knacks, stationery and greeting cards. Ali, the owner, had been an Aramco employee for many years and although he now needed neither the store nor the income he enjoyed long discussions with those of us who wandered into his domain.

He could usually be found sitting at the counter of his shop, picking his teeth with a 'toothbrush' stick and lamenting, in excellent English, the state of society and the economy.

Around the corner from the Singer store, the East West store opened battered swinging doors into a small room full of spices and other interesting foods. The heady aromas could excite even the most reluctant cook. I would hang over the half door in the back of the store and ask the attendant for scoops of various legumes, flours and spices to use in new recipes. Indian food, I discovered, was the most economical to cook and most delectable food on the planet.

You could buy any spice imaginable at the East-West store—except nutmeg. Someone had discovered that if you ate a kilogram of nutmeg you might experience a high and thus it was *haraam*, a forbidden substance. The same taboo also applied to pure vanilla essence. But even these things were available in certain places for a price.

Across the road from the East West store was a stall offering Indian *dal* and flatbread, a treat to brighten the darkest day. On the other side of town a small store constantly churned out falafels and pita sandwiches. It cost the grand sum of ten riyals, about three dollars, for an ample meal for two.

A little further on was a shop selling vegetable *samosas*, crisp triangles of flaky pastry filled with potato, peas and other vegetables in a spicy sauce. Samosas with haloumi cheese or meat were also available as a special treat during the holy month of Ramadan. Among other treats to be had were *zaatar* spices, *foul* (beans), *hommous* (chickpea dip) and the accompanying *kubs*, (flat bread).

Wheat was heavily subsidized in the Kingdom, hence one could enjoy a prepared meal in these small villages for only a few riyals.

Rahima had its share of tailors. There were many good male tailors but the Star Tailor at the end of town was different. You were only allowed behind the locked doors if you were female. The dressmaker was a Filipina who could measure and design anything, and produce a perfect fit every time.

It was rumored that some of the male tailors in town had been arrested for measuring women. Male tailors had to be content with making copies of garments, or getting lists of measurements from their customers, for it was forbidden to touch a woman no matter how innocently it was done.

One of our favorite tailors disappeared and we heard that he had been jailed for selling little white pills. He was being beaten daily as punishment for his sins.

The main street was Forty-ninth street. Here one could find electronics, grocery stores, vegetable *suqs* and carpet stores. Men did the shopping in Forty-ninth street, although expatriate women who ventured into shops here were always treated with respect.

Parallel to Forty-ninth street was Forty-seventh street, the women's street. It was lined by fabric stores on one side and gold *suqs* on the other. The walls of the *suqs* dripped with gold and there was more for sale under the counters. A large variety of westernized jewelry glittered on the shelves, as well as Saudi Arabian wedding sets—heavy earrings, bracelets, rings and huge breastplates.

"How much is that?" asked a friend once, pointing to a particularly elaborate wedding set.

"Too much for you!" replied the Indian attendant jauntily.

Gold jewelry was sold by weight rather than by the piece, cheaper here than outside the country. Although I could never figure out where most of the other forty-odd streets in Rahima were, there was enough to keep me busy every time I went to town.

The sidewalks here were all of different heights, requiring concentration to traverse without stumbling. At first I was afraid to cross the lanes of jostling traffic but soon learned that if I stepped out cautiously the traffic would stop for me.

There must have been at least fifteen mosques in Rahima. At prayer times every one of them honed their loudspeakers and competed in a cacophony of sound that was calculated to wake the conscience of even an infidel. If the wind was coming from the right direction, the prayer call could be heard across the highway in the camp.

One late afternoon I walked the borders of RT camp. The sun hung low in the sky, its last rays sparkling on Japanese grass wet from the sprinklers. As I passed the tiny mosque on the edge of the compound a solitary mellow voice broke the silence. Spellbound, I stopped to listen. The intonation was precise, the melody haunting in the traditional way of the East and I wanted to hold onto the moment forever. *That*, I said to myself, is a call to prayer.

The day the new Physical Therapy Unit in Ras Tanura opened, I waited nervously for my first patient at starting time. He arrived with a friend in tow, grinning arrogantly. His body rippled with muscles we would have killed for in the anatomy lab—a perfect specimen—but my assessment revealed that he had no more reason for treatment than I did. I thought carefully about my next move. I could not cause him to lose face but I also would not stoop to unprofessional treatment, which could set a precedent and result in an avalanche of similar cases.

"I am going to give you some exercises to do at home," I said.

"No! I want a massage." He looked cockily at his companion.

I was not to be swayed and he was the first and last patient who tried to get away with manipulating the therapist.

There was no problem filling my schedule from the start and it soon became evident that I would need help. I began to split the appointment slots on my schedule, booking two patients in at a time, and was soon literally running from patient to patient. In my previous job I had handled these numbers but, with added time for translation and the tedious paper work, there were now too many.

On top of this, there was the computer work to do each evening after the last patient had left and it was not unusual to finish work after six in the evening. It was often later than that when I wearily pedaled home on my bike.

Every employee in Aramco was expected to have a basic level of English, but in reality some had little practical ability with the language. Aramco also provided medical care for dependents of employees, and many of these spoke no English at all. Although I had all the cheat sheets Malouf had made up for me, and knew how to ask all the right questions, I often had trouble understanding the answers. I needed an assistant who could translate!

"We'll lend you a Physical Therapy assistant from Dhahran for mornings," James said, "until we find a full-time assistant for you."

Daniel was a Filipino, short in stature and quiet by nature, but I quickly learned that he was an expert in everything to do with rehabilitation in Aramco, and a rock to lean on.

It was a great day, though, when I got my own full-time helper. James called me with the good news.

"He is a Physical Therapy assistant, and can double as a receptionist," he said.

"Great!" I exclaimed. "When can he start?"

"He's ready now," said James. "He's going to be good for this job I think. He is an Arab, but he and his parents lived in the USA for ten years from the time he was four years old so his English is excellent."

Suheim was short, a little plump, and very cheerful. He wrung my hand in a firm handshake and won my heart immediately with a grin that lit up the room.

4 - OUT AND ABOUT IN AL KHOBAR

SAUDI ARAMCO OPERATES four family camps in the Eastern Province. Dhahran is the administrative center and the largest complex; Ras Tanura is an hour away and north of Dhahran, while Abqaiq is an hour to the south and Udhailiyah is another hour further south. These four camps are known as the 'quad area'.

Buses ran between Ras Tanura and Dhahran every hour during the week, and less frequently on a weekend which, in Saudi Arabia, is Thursday and Friday. Buses also took shoppers to the towns of Al-Khobar, Rahima and Dammam. From Ras Tanura, a shopping trip to either Dammam or Khobar could be an all-day experience.

If you were caught in town at prayer time, you had two choices. You could wait outside somewhere, trying to look inconspicuous if you were a female, or you could rush into a restaurant and order lunch. If you chose the latter option you were virtually a prisoner, though a well-fed one, until prayer time was over and the doors were unlocked.

At certain restaurants an attendant would let you in or out through a passage into a side alley, after checking that the coast was clear of *mutawas*, religious police, on the prowl. However, generally you had to plan your shopping trip and lunch around prayer time.

Customer service is taken very seriously in the Middle East. Many storekeepers give cups of tea to customers to sip on as they browse. If you are on foot, a shopkeeper will hold your purchases for you until you finish for the day and return to collect them. One day a shopkeeper spotted me coming and ran down the street, bringing me my purchases from his store.

I had been in Kingdom just a short time when I walked past an oriental carpet store. A beautiful carpet on a wall in the shop caught my attention, and I stopped. The Indian attendant called out to me.

"Come in! Just have a look!"

"No, no," I answered. "I am not buying carpets today, thank you."

"That's OK. Just come and look. No problem."

I succumbed, walked in and examined the carpet more carefully. It certainly was a fine piece of work, but I'd been doing an excellent job of resisting temptation until my debts were paid off and I had no intention of breaking down now.

"I'll take it down and you can look at it on the floor," the Indian offered.

"No, really! I told you I am not interested today," I said. "Although it is a lovely carpet."

But the carpet was already down and I was powerless to stop myself circling it, admiring the subtle color changes as the light fell on the grain at different angles.

"Take it home," the storekeeper said. "No need to pay for it now. Just take it home and look at it. If you like it, you can bring the money back, and if you don't like it, just bring it back here again."

"You can't just let someone take a carpet home!" I was aghast.

"Why not? Take it! You will see if it suits your house. No need to buy it if you don't want."

"Don't you want my ID number? My name?"

"No need!" The Indian's head wobbled like Jello.

I wrote my contact details down anyway, then staggered out with the carpet I loved but couldn't afford rolled up under my arm. The Indians knew what they were doing. It was impossible to part with the carpet. A week later I was back in the store with the money.

On a corner of King Khalid Street, in the centre of Al Khobar, stood an antique store. The ground floor offered treasures from Asia—wooden elephants, hand carved screens, Russian samovars, gold embroidered Damascus tablecloths, alabaster and jade vases, and furniture. At the back of the room a rickety, narrow staircase led up to the floor above.

One day I ventured up it, to a room stuffed with antiques. The scent of time pervaded the place. Silver swords and daggers in filigree sheaths covered the walls and a walkway squeezed between piles of copper pots that rose like giant stalagmites, not quite touching the ceiling.

Jewelry, new and old coffee pots, camel stools, brightly colored saddlebags, and baskets from the western, mountainous area of Najran were all jammed in wherever space permitted. There were many things I had never seen before and I could have spent hours up there browsing, breathing in as I wormed my way between the dusty stacks.

I was alone, lost in another world. Except for the Arab shop owner, a tubby, middle-aged man in a dirty-white thowb, who had padded softly up the stairway behind me. At first I thought nothing of it but suddenly he was beside me, pressing his body against me, wrapping his arms around my waist.

Dismayed, I pulled away, trying to distance myself without being rude, but he was stronger than me. This was a most awkward predicament, unacceptable in any culture let alone in Saudi Arabia. Stay cool, I told myself.

"I want you to have a gift," he purred. "Choose something. Anything! It will be yours."

I tried to refuse.

"I will choose something but I want to pay for it. And I have to go now and catch my bus."

"It's all right, take something. It will be a gift for you. And when you come back next time I will give you something else."

His breath stank of garlic and his eyes were red-veined marbles. His leering mouth revealed stained teeth, with brown deposits where they met the gums.

My mind raced. I had to choose something to save face for him, but something of such low value that it would leave me without obligation. My eyes lit on a small ring with a broken stone in it. He picked it up and tucked it into my hand and I used the distraction to pull away from him and head down the stairs.

"Thank you very much!" I said. "That is very kind of you but I really have to go now because my bus is leaving."

"Where do you live?" he asked, red eyes glittering.

"Ras Tanura," I said, speeding up a little. *And I will certainly not come back here again!*

I did return, but the only other time I dared go upstairs to the floor of enchanting antiques was with a male friend. Even then, the old shopkeeper winked and pursed his lips at me in a kissing action, when my friend's back was turned. I was revolted. It was a pity, because I had loved that store.

Desert Designs was an up-market store near the Shula Mall. It also sold antiques and classy items from all over Asia which appealed to the expat population. It was a much-frequented store, with its offerings well presented. Furniture, Bedouin jewelry mounted in shadow boxes, swords, carpets, linen goods, prayer beads—there was something for everyone. Large silver coins, which had once been currency in Saudi Arabia, were also on sale. The Arabs trusted the quality of Austrian silver more than any other, and so their original coins had been Austrian.

But of all the fascinating shops in Al-Khobar, none could compare with the gold *suqs*, which glowed together along an alley off King Khalid Street. Gold jewelry was sold here by weight and came in several grades. Twenty-four carat gold was as close to pure as possible, although one could be fooled into thinking it was cheap costume jewelry—it was too 'yellow' compared with the low karat stuff most of us were used to.

Even gold crosses were available for a price if you knew where to go and asked discreetly. Bracelets and necklaces were so affordable that some women, like my friend Kathy, collected a new piece every time they went to town. Her jewelry glistened and tinkled with every move.

"I wear my gold all the time," she confided. "Even in the shower and in bed!"

If a store didn't sell what you wanted, you could easily have a piece custom-made by any of the fine goldsmiths for little more than the price of gold. Name pendants in Arabic writing were especially popular.

It was considered 'immoral' to charge import duty on anything, so items in Kingdom were usually cheaper than if you bought them in their countries of origin. Expats stocked up on gold and such things as German steel knives, cutlery, china sets and saucepans, and top-brand names in running shoes from shoe stores. There was also a store offering "Perfumes and Honey."

Bargaining was a part of life in Saudi Arabia, although I was never very good at it. If you showed interest in anything, you risked being swept into the game, and vendors were almost disappointed if you accepted the first price offered.

Large stores such as the British Home Store were not into bargaining, and I couldn't afford anything here except at sale time. Once I asked for a fitting room.

"We don't have fitting rooms," was the answer. "Too much shoplifting. You can buy the clothing and take it home. But, if it doesn't suit you, bring it back for change or a refund."

It appeared that some unscrupulous females would put clothing on and leave the store with it under their *abayas!* As only men were allowed to serve in stores and were not permitted to challenge the women, far less to search them, they were powerless to stop the shoplifting.

The Shula Mall was crowded, dirty and old. But, everybody loved it. It was a landmark which Maria and Dean had pointed out to me on my first visit to the town. You could find almost anything in the Shula Mall. The Big Apple on the upper floor was everyone's favorite store with cards, plaques, framed photos and souvenirs of all kinds. It was heartbreaking for many of us when the Shula Mall caught fire and burned down in 1999. It burned for three days, and nothing was saved. It was like losing an old friend.

Around the corner from the Shula Mall was Latif's Bakery. Here one could buy divine flatbread, filled with cheese, *zataar* spices, or pizza toppings of various kinds. There was usually a long line of customers at the counter, and it was a favorite place to stop for lunch at prayer time.

The Rashid Mall opened in 1996. It was more of a palace than a shopping centre. With marble pillars and amazing fountains it enthralled Westerners and Saudi Arabs alike.

Just after it opened, a toddler caught hold of the handrail on the escalator—while standing *outside* the escalator! She was carried up almost to the next floor, and a concerned crowd quickly gathered. Finally she lost her hold and fell. But, a security officer lunged forward and caught the tiny girl, saving her life.

No trip to Khobar was complete without a visit to Al Zamil's, near the Aramco bus stop. Two storeys, full of everything a craft lover could wish for, provided a great place to spend the last hour or so before catching the bus home. Al Zamil's had served expatriates since the conception of Aramco. Single female employees and married women (dependent wives) alike relied on Al Zamil's for craft supplies.

Other interesting stores included general shops stuffed with hardware, kitchen ware and linens. There were pharmacies, electronic stores selling watches, cameras, and every conceivable type of television and sound-producing machine, and fabric stores with all the exotic fabrics of the East.

The large, modern Safeway supermarket on the Corniche, looking out on the Arabian Gulf, provided items which were not always available in our commissaries at the compounds.

My head was usually spinning when I returned from a shopping trip to Khobar, and still in my dreams I sometimes wander its uneven streets and peer through dusty windows, hunting for a bargain that is surely there, somewhere.

5 - KIDNAPPED!

EVERY EXPATRIATE WORKER in Saudi Arabia is provided with an *iqama,* an ID document valid for travel within Kingdom, and mine had not been processed by the time my first *Eid* arrived.

Unable to travel out of the Eastern Province, I wondered what to do for the five day holiday. Almost all the other expats had gone either overseas or camping. Even my orientation mates had received their *iqamas,* in-Kingdom identification documents, by now and had sallied off to Thailand, Jordan and other exotic destinations.

I could choose to spend my time moping on the beach or I could find something else to do. Being relatively short of cash I decided to take a free Aramco shopping bus one day to the city of Dammam and explore.

The large green and white Mercedes bus was more of a luxury coach than a bus, with reclining seats, plush upholstery and air-conditioning. It was my first solo foray into unexplored territory and I felt a shiver of apprehension as I set off, the only expatriate on board.

There was little but desert to see through the large windows until we entered the city and pulled up in an empty lot near a hotel on Fifth Street. I tried to memorize the surroundings before I disappeared into the summer haze towards the town.

The *suq* area sprawled for many blocks, teasing me onwards. The feel of silken cloth, heady aromas of the spice markets, breathy murmuring of Arabian voices and a myriad of taxis honking in the background in hopes of a fare—I eagerly soaked up the new sensations.

I'd worn my *abaya* for the first time in public, but it wasn't long before I felt like throwing it off. No wonder women came into the clinic like melted butter after being out in the sun.

Thinking of women, there *were* no women around, apart from myself. I wandered several blocks before I saw three small huddles of black on a street corner. Hesitantly I approached and they rushed towards me, jabbering excitedly.

"*Salaam. Kaif halik?* Greetings. How are you?"

I responded with a phrase Malouf had taught me in a mischievous moment, "*Fowg anakl!* Top of the palm tree!"

With screams of delighted laughter they clutched at me like children, wanting to know my name, where I came from, if I was married and how many children I had—the essentials of an Arabian woman's existence. They lifted their veils briefly, giving me glimpses of merry dark eyes. Our exchange was intense but brief, for my limited Arabic was quickly exhausted, and we parted reluctantly.

Shops in Arabia were very logically arranged. When you wanted to buy shoes you went to the area where the shoe shops were. Gold *suqs* were in one area, kitchenware in another, fabrics somewhere else, and so on. It was all very sensible. If you couldn't find what you wanted in one store, the shopkeeper would obligingly point you to another store in the same block which might have it. He might even leave his store and take you there.

I moved on, crossing streets, investigating one *suq* after another until suddenly I realized I was hopelessly lost. And the time for the bus to depart was drawing close.

Every corner looked the same, the street names confusing in Arabic and English. No matter, I thought, pulling out the crumpled Aramco timetable with a map of Dammam on the back. It was a bad photocopy, lines blurred, small and difficult to read.

I pored over it, panic rising. I *must* catch the bus back to RT! It was the only bus of the day and I could not afford a taxi home. Time passed. I would have to spend ten precious riyals on a taxi to take me to the bus stop.

But where were the taxis now? I looked around in desperation. *Barp! Barp!* A white car pulled up beside me and the driver leaned forward, with a wide smile. Trembling with relief I plunged through the rear door onto cool velvet and the driver stepped on the accelerator.

"Fifth Street, please, to the Aramco bus stop," I said.

"I am single, I like you!" the driver said as he reached back and handed me the largest bag of boiled sweets I had ever seen.

Shocked, I pulled my wits about me. This was not a taxi! How could I have been so stupid as to have gotten into a vehicle that wasn't a taxi?

"I am single, I like you!" The man repeated.

He was a large man, in a non-descript *thowb*, and his smile dazzled white under a thick black moustache. I glanced out the window. A street sign flashed by, then another, and another. Now I could see numbered streets. But the driver had ignored my request. Ninth Street...Tenth Street...heck, he was taking me *away* from the bus stop!

"*Fifth* Street!" I said very firmly, beginning to perspire again. "*Khamsa!*" I held up five trembling fingers.

"I am single, I like you!" he said with another toothy grin, reaching back toward me again.

This time he produced a large bottle of sickly-sweet perfume, which he sprayed over me. Thoughts of slavery, imprisonment, rape and murder flashed through my mind. *Please God help me.*

"No! Take me to Fifth Street!" I said again, my voice cracking as Eighteenth and Nineteenth Streets disappeared behind us.

Whether it was the prompting of my guardian angel or simply the unappealing sight of my perspiring red face I do not know, but my uncooperative chauffeur suddenly sighed, slowed, turned, and began speeding back the way we had come.

A few minutes later I saw the large green and white Aramco bus parked in the empty lot I had been searching for, and heaved a sigh of relief.

"Telephone!" said the driver.

I gave him a fake number, using the correct prefix for Dhahran and any old suffix hoping that I wasn't landing some other unsuspecting female in a hornet's nest.

"Thank you very much," I said as I stepped shakily out of the car.

"I am single, I like you!" he sang again as he drove off.

And that was the end of my first trip to Dammam.

6 - WITHIN THE WALLS

"JUDY! WOULD YOU do me a favor? We're leaving for repat in a couple of weeks; can you house sit for us and look after our dogs?"

I had barely arrived in Ras Tanura and was still trying to settle in to my own accommodation.

"Ummm...OK, sure!" I answered.

Single females were greatly in demand as house sitters for families going on repatriation, or 'repat', the period of time that workers were out of Kingdom on annual leave. The theory was that the house sitter would enjoy the benefits of living in a family house for several weeks and at the same time care for pets and plants while the usual tenants were away.

I loved animals and always accepted an invitation to house sit although it was a little wearying living out of a suitcase and plastic bags. There was usually a lot more work to do in a house. Animals, however delightful, were a chore. If the animal was a dog, the job also involved cleaning up dog turds, taking the dog on long walks and undertaking dog washing sessions.

The best house sits were those where the owners had kindly kept on their houseboys for the duration of their holidays to minimize housework on my part. However it *was* pleasant to have the space to host a nice dinner party and to have room to invite friends up from Dhahran for a night or two on a weekend.

My first house sit involved caring for two terriers. One was actually the father of the other and had taken to quietly terrorizing the other at mealtimes. Dad, after finishing his own food, would march over to Sonny Boy's dish and polish that off as well. The problem worsened during my first week at the house until I wondered if the younger dog would starve to death under my charge.

One night I decided that enough was enough. I dragged the younger dog over to its bowl of food, aware of a subliminal threat coming from the older dog. Force-feeding the younger animal was not easy. He was obviously hungry but, between gulps at the food I pushed into his mouth, his eyes rolled backwards and he yelped in fear.

Satisfied that both dogs had been fed, I left the room but, a moment later, an awful commotion erupted in the kitchen. I dashed back in. Dad was snarling and snapping, straddling the younger dog which was belly-up and howling in terror. What to do? I grabbed a newspaper and thumped the aggressor repeatedly, snarling and growling myself in a manner that befitted the leader of a pack.

I was deeply thankful that nobody was around to witness this ridiculous behavior but, from that moment on the older dog accepted his place as a subordinate. There was no more bullying. Law and order had been established.

One memorable house-sit involved caring for a dog, a canary, a large parrot and an aviary with about twenty cockatiels. The instructions for each day were written on several sheets of foolscap. The dog in this case was the easiest charge, requiring only two walks and meals per day, and a weekly bath. The aviary birds were to have their water bowls cleaned and filled daily and three types of seed, as well as cooked corn. The canary was to have seed, a lettuce leaf, three cooked peas, two niblets of corn, and a piece of cooked carrot and a change of drinking water.

The large parrot lived in a cage in the garage. It was suffering from some type of brain disease which caused it to hang upside down in the cage and clamber about drunkenly. The parrot was to be given half an apple, half an orange, half a banana, a slice of bread and a scoop of ice-cream at each feeding. Getting the food to it was a test of speed and agility, for it could squirt a stream of excreta with incredible accuracy at a human target a great distance away.

It took an hour to get around the menagerie every morning. I was exhausted before I even arrived at work and was heartily relieved when the owners returned. There were no mishaps apart from one natural death (a cockatiel) and the loss of the dog for an afternoon (he had gone into the bathroom and jumped up on the door, closing himself in). A few weeks after I left, I met the lady of the house again, in the commissary.

"Hello!" I said brightly. "How are the birds and the dog doing?"

"Fine," she said. "We're making frozen yogurt for the parrot now!" I wished her luck.

Then there was the house-sit that included Fred, the basset. I loved the friendly old dog and he was easy to care for. When time came for his first weekly bath, though, I wondered how I was going to manage. He would not get into the bath tub and there was no way I could lift him. Then I remembered something. He loved chocolate! In fact, he had knocked over the Christmas tree the night before I had arrived I was told, and had eaten all the chocolates off the tree.

I knew where there was one more chocolate. I broke it in half, gave Fred one half to eat and threw the other half into the bath tub. He hesitated for a long moment then jumped in after it.

"Gotcha!" I said.

The story was told about a girl and her boyfriend, the 'house sitters from hell,' who suffered one disaster after another while caring for a house and a cat.

First, the cat escaped and was hit by a car before anybody could retrieve it. It was not killed but suffered multiple injuries and the vet bill was enormous.

Later on, an antique chair broke. The boyfriend took it to a repair shop in Dammam but, when he went to pick it up, he couldn't remember which shop he'd taken it to! Bad, bad move. He could not find a replacement for the chair.

Then the smoke detector battery died, so the boyfriend removed it. Shortly afterwards a fire demolished the kitchen, resulting in huge reconstruction bills for the company. The girl took the rap for that—the boyfriend worked for Loss Prevention and would have lost his job if he'd admitted liability.

One of my nicest house sits was in a beach house with one cat, a gentle old Persian which was strictly a house cat and had been de-clawed. I didn't even have to clean the house as the houseboy was kept on for the duration of the householders' vacation. All I had to do was to keep the cat's litter box clean, feed her, and give her hairball medicine and lots of attention. Easy! The gentle sound of the surf lulled me to sleep every night, and mornings came with soft pastel views over the sea.

One day the cat was not in evidence as per normal. Thinking she may be hiding somewhere, I checked every room and every cupboard, calling her name. No luck. It's possible I missed her the first time, I thought, and decided to search again. By the third search I was getting hot and cold chills. Had she slipped through my legs when I shook out the tablecloth? Had I unwittingly left a window open? Thoughts of the house-sitters from hell began to haunt me. This cat was not just a cat; she was part of the family.

On my hundredth pass through the house I came to the kitchen and happened to look up. There, sitting innocently on top of the refrigerator and staring down at me curiously, was the cat! Truly, I thought, dogs come when you call, but cats take a message and get back to you.

I felt a bit sorry for old Tiny, Chad and Naomi Anderson's dog.

"He only needs to be walked once a day," they told me cheerfully before leaving on repat. "If you're a bit late back from work in the afternoon you'll find him crossing his legs though."

That was a bit of a worry—sometimes I did not get back from work until rather late.

I couldn't help myself; I had to take him out twice a day to sniff the grass and have a pee and the big black poodle was ecstatic. However the consequences of my generosity did not become apparent until Tiny's owners returned.

"I think his bladder has shrunk," said Chad glumly when I next saw him. "It'll probably take some time to stretch it out again!"

One morning at work I learned that a British patient's wife was arriving the next week and staying for a month. He worked in a male compound and did not have family status, so depended on house sits for accommodation when his wife came into Kingdom.

Men on the British payroll had to have a certain grade code level before they were allowed family status. Those without family status were granted more leave than those with families, and their wives were also permitted to come into Kingdom for a few months each year, if their husbands could find house-sits for them.

"I don't know what to do," he said. "I had a house sit lined up, but it has fallen through, and I have nowhere for my wife to stay when she arrives."

I wanted to help him out. I had a house-sit myself, for the exact dates he needed, but a sense of honesty jerked me back from offering it to him. The man seemed awfully nice. I still, however, could not feel comfortable passing on the trust which had been placed in me.

Then a sudden thought struck me—he and his wife could stay in *my* house! He was delighted with the offer and loved my apartment. It was quite big enough for two and when their time ended it was exactly as I'd left it—with the addition of a large bunch of flowers and a thank-you card.

Occasionally I enjoyed a swim in the Gulf, especially when house-sitting for someone in a beach house. The bay was generally a comfortable temperature and it was relaxing to snorkel out to the man-made reef and watch the fish. There, where coral grew abundantly over things like old engine blocks and roof racks, the snap and crackle of fish feeding sounded like eggs frying.

The two men who had established the reef still lived on camp and sometimes dragged even more old hardware out to extend it. Rays, anemones and many tropical fish thrived here as well as the odd small shark. Friends who came for a sleepover and a snorkel never forgot the experience. Living here was a world apart, and everything was so easy.

7 - LIFE IN THE ARAMCO LANE

I SLIPPED ON A baggy shirt and some long pants and checked the bus timetable. A bus to Rahima was due to leave the mail centre at nine o'clock and I could do my errands and be home before noon prayers.

At the Rahima pharmacy, three young Arabian women were trying on sunglasses. One would place a pair on her face, over her veil and head scarf, while the other two nodded or shook their heads, as if trying to imagine what their friend would look like in the glasses and helping with her decision.

A visit to the bank was next on my list. As I entered, the men in line at the counter all fell back. I paused, stunned, as the teller motioned for me to approach the counter. Once again I was served first, simply because I was a woman.

I needed to see the bank manager about a check and was soon in deep discussion with him. Abdul Al Mota was a gentle man with a swarthy complexion and a dark patch in the center of his forehead, which I later discovered was a thickened area due to much pressing of the head to the floor during prayer rituals.

Abdul's English was poor and he desperately wanted to improve it. "Can I come to your house for one hour every week to speak English with you?" he asked.

I hesitated. It seemed wrong somehow, allowing a Saudi Arabian male to enter my home when their own rules of etiquette demanded complete separation of male and female populations. According to an Arabian proverb, 'If a man and a woman are alone in one place, the third person present is Satan'.

Yet Abdul seemed honest and his desperation to improve his language skills swayed me.

"OK," I said finally, "I'll be home most evenings."

And so began my association with him and his delightful family. He was always a gentleman, staying only an hour each time he came and engaging only in English conversation. His English did improve, although his accent became distinctly Australian as time went on.

At work, the referrals were pouring in. Physical Therapy policy instructed therapists to take only three new patients a day, as well as those with follow-up appointments. I was taking many more. This meant that follow-up appointments had to be spaced further apart to allow more patients to fit into my schedule. Home programs became more important, getting patients to take more responsibility for their conditions. James called me from the Dhahran clinic.

"You'll have to stop taking so many patients—you're showing the rest of us up!"

"But they just keep coming," I said. "What can I do? I can't send them away."

"Start a waiting list. Prioritize. Tell people you'll call them in as soon as you get an available slot and keep strictly to only three new patients a day."

Some patients accepted the inevitable wait for treatment graciously. Others insisted on immediate treatment and created a great disturbance at Reception if they were put off. Although I couldn't always understand the Arabic that Suheim used, I drew comfort from his dulcet tones in the background as I worked, knowing that nine times out of ten the anger would subside and the patient would walk away satisfied, if not smiling.

Once in a while he would call me in desperation and I would go to reception with a sinking heart. Sometimes it would have been quicker to bring the patient in for treatment then and there than to argue, for I would end up with a backlog of people in the waiting area before the issue was settled.

As a last resort I tried a method James had suggested—showing the schedule to the patient and asking which of the others on the list he would like me to bump so that he could have that slot. Invariably he would be horrified at the thought and reluctantly accept his fate on the waiting list. Something in the culture precluded a person from taking the place of another.

I often wondered about the two sharply distinct types of patient—those who accepted whatever they were offered with an "*Inshallah* (God willing)," and those who argued their case loudly and unrelentingly.

It was an Arabian physical therapy student who explained it to me.

"The strong-headed ones are desert people. They are used to fighting against the desert for their lives and they have to be strong to exist against the weather, the heat and the sand. They are tough and when they come to town or to the clinic, they are still fighting."

I had to admire their spirit even if it wore me down at times. Yet it was not only the Bedouin who could be difficult at the reception window. The occasional expatriate stood up to the receptionist as fiercely as the most ardent desert dweller.

The first few months passed in rather a blur. Several people were anchors for me in my new job and one was Navi, a Sri Lankan man who was the glue that held everyone together, or so it seemed. If I had a problem, a question, or just wanted to chat, he was there. It seemed there was nothing he couldn't do and he had contacts everywhere.

Some months after arriving in RT, I bought a piano from a lady in Dhahran. It was a very good price and seemed like a gift from heaven. Bringing it home to Ras Tanura was a problem and I asked if Navi could help by recommending someone with a truck.

"How much will it cost to move the piano?" I wondered.

Navi smiled.

"Let's ask the friends first!" he said.

Someone owed him a favor and it would not cost a penny. Several of his friends accompanied us to

Dhahran. The men wrestled the piano onto the truck and it was delivered to my apartment free of charge.

The men shuffled the piano into a niche along a wall in my living room. It was a wall connecting my apartment with a neighbor's and I asked Jim if he could hear the piano through the wall, as I did not want to disturb him.

"A piano! I did think I heard something," he said, "though it was very faint. I could barely hear it at all."

Reassured, I continued to play the piano without fear of disturbing him unduly. And a few weeks later when I woke up early one morning, I thought nothing of tinkling the ivories a little. At ten minutes to seven as I left for work, I noticed a yellow post-it note clamped to my front door.

"Please do not play the piano at 5 am," it read. "6 am yes. 5 am no." It was signed, Jim Baker.

I felt a stab of dismay—I had annoyed my neighbor! How inconsiderate he must think me. It bothered me all day, and when I bumped into Jim at the mail centre my first thought was to apologize. But he got in first.

"Did you get my note this morning?" he asked peevishly.

"Yes," I said, "I thought you couldn't hear me as I'd asked you early on and you said you could hardly hear the piano. I'm so sorry. I'm really, *really* sorry!"

Jim stood speechless. Perhaps he had expected me to become aggressive and defensive rather than apologetic.

A week or so later, the phone rang.

"I suppose you'll think this is funny," he said sheepishly, "but I'd like you to play the piano for me."

It seemed that he had a rather good voice and had received an invitation to sing a couple of golden oldies at a function in a few weeks' time. I agreed to record an accompaniment for him if he provided me with the music and we enjoyed some practice sessions together before the event.

"Casual" employees filled a number of positions on camp. Casuals were married women who held jobs as regular employees did but for much lower wages, as their husbands were considered the primary employees and received the family benefits.

Amanda was one of these casual employees, a petite American with dark curls and alabaster skin. She was the receptionist in the X-ray unit at the time and took me under her wing, giving me advice and assistance like a kind aunt. During the first months, hardly a day went by that Amanda didn't stop to visit and give me something tasty to augment my lunch. She will never know how many times her little gift *was* my lunch!

Another option for lunch was the 'roach coach,' a van that came at a certain time every day. Pig products are forbidden in the Moslem religion, so the burgers were called "*hum*burgers," so as not to be confused with anything containing pork.

Other foods were available, and I usually got an egg sandwich. One day I was embarrassingly short of cash when I opened my purse to pay for my lunch. An Arabian man behind me thrust a ten riyal note into my hand and brushed off my thanks with a wave of his hand.

"You must tell me where you work," I insisted, "I'll pay you back!"

"No need," he said with a shrug and a smile. It was one of many times I experienced Saudi Arabian generosity and hospitality.

8 - OUT IN THE SANDPIT

ONE DAY ON the weekend, shortly after moving to Ras Tanura, I walked the dogs in the late morning. It was my first house sit, the one with the two terriers, and I was determined to do a good job.

After I returned from the walk the phone rang. It was an unfamiliar voice, that of a man who introduced himself as Rob and asked me if I would have lunch with him. It was an American voice I thought, and sounded courteous enough. My first thought was to politely refuse but then I thought—why not? Nothing could happen to me on the compound and it might be a pleasant interlude.

I discovered that one of my patients had called Rob, who'd been divorced for some years, and told him that he really should meet the new physical therapist on camp. She described me, and at that instant he saw me walk past his window with the two dogs! He recognized the dogs. After he'd given me time to finish the walk, he looked up the phone number of his friends who owned the dogs.

Rob was of average build, about three inches taller than I and with blue-grey eyes, prominent nose and fair hair beginning to grey. His voice was quiet and polite, and he had what I learned was a Canadian accent.

Lunch was simple, just toasted sandwiches, and we shared information about ourselves and why we'd come to work in Aramco. It was a friendly but not scintillating encounter and as I left the house I thought it would be the last. However, one day after work, Rob called again.

"I'm going camping on the weekend," he said. "There's another Australian couple going and I thought perhaps you'd like to come too. We're going to drive west of Riyadh to a large crater in a remote area."

I paused to consider. The camping trip would be a wonderful opportunity. Unfortunately, it fell during another house-sit commitment and I was reluctant to pass over the responsibility I'd accepted. However after some persuasion I agreed to find someone else to feed the cat for the few days we'd be away, and allowed myself to become excited about the coming long weekend.

The *Wabah* Crater trip was the beginning of a grand adventure in Kingdom. I never felt more freedom in my life than when we set out in Rob's old Land Cruiser. Armed with our *iqamas* and letters of permission from the company, we trundled out along highways and sandy tracks, and when there were no more tracks we made our own.

We could pinpoint our position accurately with a GPS, or, global positioning system, and never be completely lost. Fences were almost non-existent and when we came across Bedou, nothing more serious than an invitation to tea and dates ever hampered us.

Evenings camping in the desert were cool. We spent hours sitting around campfires talking, laughing, and watching the flames. The Australian couple entertained us with stories of their experiences prospecting for arrowheads. When we retired to our cots in the open air I would lie on my back, staring at the stars that pricked the black sky until my eyes blurred.

Mornings brought hot oatmeal and early departures, with long days in a desert that gradually changed from flat plains in the Eastern Province to spectacular escarpments around Riyadh, to the red sands of the Ad Dhana and then rough tracks through rocky terrain and stumpy shrubs. Small hills swelled along the horizon as we neared our target.

"Care should be taken when approaching the crater," I read from the photocopied sheets we had been given. "You will reach the crater before you see it. If you are going too fast you will plummet over the edge before your passengers can query your parentage."

The crater was breathtakingly immense. It was over eight hundred feet deep and more than a mile across, with a striking white floor which we learned was salt.

According to some scientists, a gigantic gas explosion had blown the material out of this hole in the ground many years previously. We set up our camp on a ledge alongside the crater and awakened to a million-dollar view.

After breakfast there was time to go walking down the steep track to the floor of the crater. Halfway down a small grove of palms sheltered a colony of goats. Walking across the saltpan at the bottom of the path was like walking on a spongy trampoline. Names had been carved into the salt crust; the writing would disappear after the next rain.

My first camping trip had given me a whole new perspective on Arabia and I longed for more. After that I took every available opportunity to go camping with Rob. We also found ourselves meeting frequently on weekends, after work, and joining groups on extended holidays.

Desert travel was really only feasible during the cooler months, from October through April, as summer temperatures endangered both vehicle performance and lives. We traveled in groups with at least two vehicles in case of mishap. It was essential to plan carefully for desert travel and each vehicle would head out loaded up with food, spare parts and bedding, as well as fuel and plenty of water.

One day we were invited to a *kabsa*, a traditional Saudi Arabian meal. We sat cross-legged around a huge platter on the ground. The platter was filled with rice, yellowed with jasmine and smelling deliciously of Middle-Eastern spices. Portions of chicken, cooked with the rice and seasoned with the same spices, lay atop the mound.

Our host took a handful of rice, squeezed it expertly in his right palm and flicked it into his mouth, losing barely a grain. I tried to copy him but my rice ball fell apart in a hundred fragments and tumbled onto the ground. Everyone chuckled.

"You'll get used to it," Rob said. "It takes practice."

Then our host tore off a small piece of meat and flung it onto the pile of rice in front of me.

"Take it," Rob whispered. "It's custom to throw choice pieces of meat to the guests."

Meeting Bedou out in the desert was the best way to learn the customs of Saudi Arabia. Three cups of tea or coffee is polite; when you've had enough, shake your cup or turn it upside down to let your host know. Never, ever, point your foot toward someone, and use only your right hand when eating (the left is used for other, less-polite purposes). You are permitted to ask your host about his children but never to ask about his wife, especially if you are male.

Socializing is a major part of Saudi Arabian culture and even when you are in a hurry it is considered rude to rush into business without first exchanging protracted greetings and cups of hot beverage. We Westerners have lost much in our helter-skelter society, where such small courtesies are often forgotten.

One day I went with Rob to visit one of his Saudi Arabian co-workers at his home in Jubail, a port city north of our compound. The home was huge—four large apartments in all. Salim's widowed mother lived in one apartment, Salim lived in another with his wife and family, and two other brothers lived in the remaining apartments with their families.

Salim, being the oldest male, was the natural head of the family. On occasion the families would combine for meals, with women and men in their respective areas. The women spoke only Arabic. It was a challenge to converse with the women as I sat with them in the women's quarters.

"How long have you been married?" asked the old lady.

I gulped. Although I am not in the habit of lying, I wanted to save my hostess from embarrassment. In her culture it would have been unthinkable for a single woman and a single man to travel anywhere together.

And so I said, "Oh, about four years."

"How many children do you have?" another woman asked eagerly.

"None," I said truthfully, looking at a sea of concerned faces.

"That woman over there had problems getting pregnant too," someone said. "She went to a specialist hospital in Jeddah, and look—she has a child now! Why don't you do the same?"

"That sounds like a very good idea." I tried to sound enthusiastic.

Fortunately the conversation then turned to subjects that stretched the mind rather than the truth. We ate together in the women's dining room and only when it was time to leave for home was I ushered out to the men's majlis where Rob waited.

Salim wanted to go on a camping trip some day.

"I am Saudi Arabian," he told Bob, "but although my ancestors were Bedou, I don't know as much about camping in the desert as you do!"

Rob invited him along on a trip to a popular cave, *Wadi Sabsab*. Boy scouts from the compounds frequently went there on excursions as it was an interesting system to crawl around in and yet hard to get lost in. A geologist from camp also came with us.

We drove for several hours, boring into the red rocky heart of the Eastern Province, and were almost onto the opening of the cave, or *dahl*, before we saw it. The small hole was flush with the desert plain. I marveled at the accuracy of the GPS in leading us to it.

Salim eyed the hole in the ground curiously. Saudi Arabs do not generally go into holes in the ground. They are raised to have deep respect, even fear, for caves. It must have taken a great deal of courage for Salim to swallow his concerns and follow us. He was game for anything and had perfect trust in his colleague.

There were no spectacular formations here, just a challenging maze of crazy tunnels through which we spiraled downward until finally we sat triumphantly on the clay floor and took photos of each other.

That night we ate stew, told stories around the campfire, and fell asleep in our respective cots under the blazing stars. Salim was reluctant to see the end of the weekend and was keen to come again some time.

Many Saudi Arabians could not understand the purpose of going anywhere except to visit someone.

"Why do you want to go to the desert?" a patient asked once. "There's nobody there!"

Only one old patient of mine understood my keenness to travel.

"I like to travel also, not only to visit people but just to see what is there. Did you know that there is a Jewish town in the west of the country? Not many people know about it. I went there once, just to see it."

It was refreshing to find an old Arab who was so knowledgeable about his country.

One of my early trips in the desert with Rob was to the Riyadh escarpment, with several other vehicles. On the last day, we broke off from the main group and drove down to the plains. Here we spent most of the day looking for fossilized shells and other items left behind by the sea, thousands of years previously. Worried that we may not get back to camp before dark, we stopped at a Bedou camp to ask if the road ahead led back up the escarpment.

Several men were sitting on a mat in front of a cluster of tents and invited us to join them for coffee. They insisted that one of them take our photograph with the group, using my camera.

Everyone's attention turned toward the man with my camera and, taking advantage of the distraction, a man behind me reached around my shoulder and began to grope me. I swiftly twisted away and pretended that nothing had happened. It sickened me, all the same.

After the photo shoot one of the men asked if I would like to visit their women. Behind another tent several young girls stood around a very old lady, dressed in an old shift and seated on a cushion. She appeared to be blind and wore no veil.

"*Sura! Sura!* Photo! Photo!" the girls begged.

I was a little reluctant at first, knowing the restrictions many Muslims have about photographing women, but they persisted. All of them wanted their photos taken.

"Should I take her photo too?" I asked, motioning to the old woman. "She won't mind?"

"*Laa!* No!" they chorused. "*Sura! Sura!* Take a picture!"

I happily obliged. Then my guide pointed to another couple of men, who had a sheep suspended by the back legs at the back of a tent. They beckoned me to take more photos as they slit the sheep's throat and drained its blood into a bowl. It submitted silently to the assault on its life, as is the nature of sheep. After killing the sheep, the men proceeded to skin it and cut it into pieces. It was a rare opportunity to capture the essence of Bedouin life.

One of the Arabs was visiting from town and he gave us his address so I could send copies of my photographs to the group.

We had to leave soon if we wanted to get up the escarpment before dark. Our new friends gave us handfuls of sheep cheese to take with us. These hard yellow chunks smelled like dried vomit and my stomach began to turn as I bit into one. After we were far from the camp I opened the window wide and threw the cheese away.

One beautiful weekend I set off with Rob and his friend Chad to an area north east of Riyadh to search for more *dahls*, or caves. Three of my friends came with us—Tanya, Amy and Donna, who were excited at the prospect of a camping holiday. We made a stop in Rahima to pick up some fresh, hot Arab bread and *labneh*, thick yoghurt, for a breakfast 'on the road', and then headed north.

Most of the caves were in an area north-east of Riyadh, a good seven or eight hour drive from Ras Tanura. The route was tortuous after leaving the highway and Rob's old four wheel drive vehicle bucked and rattled until I was sure that it was about to split clean in half. Chad's vehicle followed well behind to avoid our dust.

Around the *dahls* were only narrow tracks, which the locals had created by criss-crossing the sandy gravel in their small pickups. It pays to follow these tracks as much as possible unless proceeding with extreme caution, as you can be upon—or into—a *dahl* before you know it.

Rain had fallen a few weeks previously. The desert had the appearance of rich pastureland; grass and flowers were knee-high and the camels were in heaven. Tiny, Chad's dog, was with him.

"I never bring food for him when we go camping," said Chad. "He doesn't bother to eat."

However Tiny was looking decidedly hungry when we began to prepare our evening meal, so I hard-boiled an egg, peeled it and passed it to Chad, who was deep in conversation with Rob.

"This is for Tiny," I said.

I looked away but turned back again in time to see Chad popping the last of the egg into his mouth.

"Chad!" I shrieked, to everyone's amusement. "That egg wasn't for you, it was for Tiny!"

Chad rolled his eyes.

"Sorry," he said, "I wasn't listening."

I cooked another egg for Tiny and gave it to the hungry dog myself.

There were many 'sinkholes' in this area, small caves and holes in the limestone substrate to explore. Some actually sported a stalactite or two but most were just holes. Still, it was fun to hunt for them, explore them and then take GPS location points on them. There was always the hope that one would prove to be a *real* cave.

In an area where a cave had collapsed we discovered a moderately high vertical cliff face and here Rob decided that Tanya and I should learn to rappel. He measured out some ropes which he attached to the Land Cruiser, made a simple harness, and explained how to descend over the edge of the cliff. I was petrified but the men assured me that the whole experience would be fun and perfectly safe.

Once over the edge I was not so sure—and all of a sudden I was upside down! Peals of laughter from below greeted this event and I was informed that this position was quite normal, in fact to be expected, in someone from 'down under'. What to do? I could panic, which would not help at all, or I could think my way through.

By wriggling and squirming I managed to right myself, but now my shirt, which was of an utterly inappropriate style for this activity, had become twisted in the rope and I was torn between fear for my ultimate safety and embarrassment lest the shirt should come completely off me.

Slowly I inched downwards, feeling a burning sensation as the rope cut into my side. Finally, with a sigh of relief, I felt my trembling feet touch terra firma, and the people who I had once thought were my friends helped me out of my harness.

Now it was Tanya's turn. With much laughter she got herself into the harness and backed carefully over the cliff edge. As I watched from the other side of the ravine she began to swing. Suddenly, her head struck a rock and she stopped moving. A trickle of blood ran down the cliff.

"No!" I cried, horrified.

They've killed her, I thought. Rob slowly lowered Tanya to the ground with the safety line he had attached to her harness.

"I'm OK," she protested as we rushed to her side. "Really! I just bumped my head and was trying to figure out how to stop swinging around."

Her yellow T shirt was drenched with blood, as was her face and hair.

"Take a photo," said someone. "We'll send it to her parents!"

And so went our first lessons in the fine art of rappelling.

On the way home we noticed a white pick-up in the distance. Only Arabs were allowed to own pick-ups. It was illegal for an expat to own one—he might use it for business purposes, which would be considered a conflict of interest to his sponsoring company.

As the pick-up drew closer we saw three young Arabs inside, dressed in white *thowbs*. They grinned at the sight of girls in the vehicles and began to show off. Their little pick-up spun around in the soft sandy soil of the *subkha*, passed us, dropped back then drove in circles again off the track.

We laughed and kept on driving, straddling the tiny striped bitter melons which grew on straggly vines between the ruts. After we had passed the boys in the pickup for about the third time, I looked back. The pickup was not moving.

"Hey! I think they're in trouble," I said.

"Are you sure?" asked Rob.

"Yes!"

We turned around. Chad followed in his car. Sure enough, the little white pick-up was well and truly stuck—right to the axles. The front wheels bit deeper and deeper into the *subkha*, boggy ground, as the driver fruitlessly continued to rev the engine.

"They must be lads from town," Rob said as he pulled up. "Bedou would never have gotten into this mess."

The young men had no recovery gear with them. Rob found a steel cable in the back of the Land Cruiser and hooked it to his bumper, then onto the pick-up. Then he turned to me with a wink.

"You pull them out," he said.

I hesitated. To drive off-road was one thing, but I had never pulled anybody out of a bog before. And it would be doubly embarrassing for the young men to be pulled out of the *subkha* by a woman!

"I'll try," I said at last.

I scrambled into the driver's seat and turned the key. Gears in reverse...easy on the accelerator...BANG! The cable had pulled off its attachment on our vehicle. Rob found a shovel and had the young men dig the boggy sand out from under the front wheels of their truck before we tried again.

This time, the white pick-up eased slowly out of its muddy prison and climbed onto firm ground. Cheers went up and I sighed with relief.

As we rolled up the cable, the young Arabian driver sidled up to me, his head hanging.

"Thank you very much!" he said sheepishly.

9 - FORBIDDEN LOVE

A YOUNG ARABIAN GIRL worked in the X-ray department as an assistant. She was strikingly beautiful, with fair skin and green eyes. Stubbornly defying tradition, she refused to wear the cloying black abaya and veil; she chose instead the simple flowing white gown and headscarf worn by Jordanian and Palestinian women.

One day, while waiting at an Aramco bus stop, she fell into conversation with one of the young American engineers. Brad was captivated by the lovely girl.

"Where are you from?" he asked.

"From here—I am a Saudi," she answered.

"Oh, I'm sorry!" he replied, stunned. "I guess I shouldn't be speaking with you then."

"It's all right," she said.

And there began a friendship that rapidly escalated into love. Brad became a Moslem to win Mariam's hand, for only a Moslem man is allowed to marry a Moslem girl. This ensures that the children will be brought up in the Moslem faith, for a man has the jurisdiction over his household.

Mariam's parents were reluctant to consider Brad at first, but he was persistent and finally won their trust and approval.

Kathy was a good friend of Brad's and helped to arrange several clandestine meetings for them at lunchtimes in her apartment. Mariam would make her way directly to the apartment while Brad entered by an adjoining building and took a devious route so nobody would see them together.

Imagine Brad's shock when, while in Bahrain one weekend, he overheard a couple of drunken Arabs discussing the fact that an American engineer was meeting a Saudi Arabian girl in secret for lunch on the Aramco compound! That was the end of the planned visits, for they could not risk being caught. The penalties for their innocent rendezvous would have been very severe.

Much as Brad loved Mariam, it was difficult arranging the marriage. The wedding and the dowry were going to be very costly and there were social obligations he had to fulfill, as well as becoming a Moslem.

As time proceeded, Brad's feet began to cool off considerably. When he met a vivacious young English woman at a party in my apartment one evening, it was the beginning of the end for Mariam. He finally told her the wedding was off.

She was devastated. Besides loving Brad, she regarded him as her ticket out of Saudi Arabia. She would not entertain the thought of marrying a Saudi

Arabian man. She had once been engaged to an Arabian, who had betrayed her and her family's trust and abused her.

Some months after Brad broke the engagement, Mariam escaped from Saudi Arabia. She told her father that she wanted to join her brother in Chicago, where he was studying. She wanted to do another course in x-ray technology.

He agreed to let her go to the care of her brother, but it was a ruse on Mariam's part. A radiology group in California had offered her a job so she slipped away to a new life. She later met and married an American and had three beautiful children.

10 - TYING THE KNOT, SHIITE STYLE

THE PHONE RANG in my apartment. It was Kathy.

"Judy! Would you like to come to a Saudi wedding with me?"

"*What?* What d'you mean? You can't just invite me to someone else's wedding!"

"Yes I can! One of the guys in the office is getting married and he's handed out a bunch of invitations. We're all going and I've got a spare one for you. Don't you want to come? It would be a great chance for you to experience a Saudi wedding."

The wedding was scheduled for 8:30 pm on a Thursday night. Three expatriate women—Kathy, Marlene, and I—clambered into Kathy's boss's car and he drove us to the wedding hall in Qatif.

The men's party was at another venue; none of the men who were invited to this wedding would ever see the bride or her attendants.

The women's hall was full of guests by the time we arrived, perhaps five hundred of them, already heavily into celebrating. We were apparently special guests and were ushered to front row seats. A raised platform at the front of the room was the dance stage, where an all-female band pounded out Middle Eastern music at a deafening volume. It was almost impossible to have a conversation.

Some women wore garments from the top fashion houses of Europe, some remained fully veiled and clad in their abayas, and others chose to dress somewhere between these extremes. Even now in Arab society, I'd heard, there were wives who even refused to completely expose themselves to their husbands.

As the crowd jostled and swayed to the music, one large figure caught my attention. She put all her energies into the dance but it was obvious that exercise was not something she was accustomed to. From time to time her immense body would crumple to the floor. The music would stop and friends would cluster about, fanning her face until she could stagger to her feet and begin dancing again. Whether the woman had a medical condition or was just overheated I could not know. I prayed that there would not be a death before the night was out.

It was almost midnight when a cry went out over the loudspeakers. The guests reacted instantly, rushing for their abayas and tying their veils about their heads.

"What's happening?" I asked.

"The bride and groom are coming," said Marlene disdainfully. "All this palaver because one man is coming into the room and might see their faces."

Suddenly the hall erupted with a shrill trilling sound, which I had never heard before. Ululation is performed by women in the Middle East when they are excited or happy, and the effect of five hundred women all doing it at once was spine-tingling.

Then the doors opened to reveal the just-married couple. The young man, clad in a black western suit, walked down the long aisle beside his bride who shimmered in a glitter of white tulle and beaded satin. Fragile and childlike, her eyes blackened with *kohl,* she looked more desperate than radiant. Several small girls, in replicas of the bridal dress, traipsed along behind.

"Gawd!" whispered Kathy. "She's only sixteen and she looks scared to death."

"She's older than a lot of brides in this country though," I reminded her, thinking of an elderly patient who had married when he was twelve and his bride eleven.

The newlyweds sat for an hour in throne-like armchairs on the platform, submitting to official photographs by a female photographer also clad in black. Then they stood and walked out through a back door.

A rumble began in the great hall. It increased in volume until I saw that the women had begun to stampede.

"What's happening?" I asked, this time concerned for *our* health.

"It's the reception," said Marlene dryly. "Better hurry or you won't get anything to eat."

The three of us eased into the flow and were swept through a wide doorway into the reception hall where three smiling attendants were waiting for us.

They handed us food-laden plates and a motley assortment of cutlery, then directed us toward three chairs at a long table. Marlene sniffed.

"It seems I'll have to eat with a knife," she said. "That's all I have."

"I'm sorry," I said, "I can't help; I only have a spoon!"

Kathy had a fork so perhaps there had only been the one setting of cutlery available and the attendants had shared it out amongst the three of us.

"I might go and get some chicken," said Kathy. "They didn't give me any."

I'd only taken about three bites of my meal before she returned.

"There isn't anything left," she said.

"Those three attendants knew what they were doing," muttered Marlene. "If it weren't for them we'd probably have starved."

"What?" I exclaimed. "Surely there must be something! I'll go and look for you."

The hall reminded me of a scene from Hitchcock's movie, "The Birds". Figures clad in voluminous black robes were perched everywhere—on tables, under tables and in the aisles. They were indeed consuming the last of the food. None of the large serving dishes had anything left in them.

One woman was scooping the last of the rice from a cauldron with her dinner plate, others were shoveling rice and meat into their mouths with their fists and one, seated at the end of our table, was picking the eyes from a sheep's skull.

Then I spied it. Dessert! Large trays of puddings stood on tables beyond the crowds. I'll get some before the masses arrive, I thought smugly.

But then I saw a dark-robed figure carrying a serving spoon from the middle of a tray to her toothless mouth. *Slurp!* She dropped the spoon back into the dish and moved on to the next tray to repeat the performance. I screeched to a halt, did an about-turn and returned to my seat.

"You're right, Kathy," I said. "There's nothing left."

11 - THE FIRST KING

ALLAHU AKHBAR! Allahu Akhbar! The melodic, breathy tones of the call to prayer floated over the rooftops, echoing through the sultry air to the red dunes and beyond.

Now the sun was sliding from the sky like a huge bowl of blood, spilling itself along the horizon. Soon it would fall beyond Arabia's shroud of sand-dust and humidity and the day would be gone.

The old mud brick buildings of Dir'aiyah, on the outskirts of Riyadh, gleamed before me in the last of the golden light. Palms nodded gently at the entrance and I gazed, fascinated, as I thought of the famous king who had once lived within these walls.

Prince Abdul Aziz Ibn Saud was born here around the year 1880 AD (by the Gregorian calendar). At that time, the palace in the city centre was surrounded by other stone-and-mud buildings, which crowded along narrow streets.

Thousands of years previously, subterranean forces had folded the crust of the earth and forced it upward creating *Wadi Hanifa*, a rift which became the western border of the city. Underground springs fed date palms and vegetable gardens nearby; *Riyadh* means "the Garden City," and was the pride of central Arabia.

Sarah, the young Abdul Aziz's mother, had been kept veiled and secluded since she was seven years of age. She was ignorant of the outside world. However, she was rich in common sense, and had much influence with her husband and children.

Until Abdul Aziz was weaned, he spent all of his time in the hareem at the palace with his mother and sister, Nura. Then he was placed under the care of a large black slave, who became his friend and personal bodyguard. The slave boys around him were also his friends.

Abdul Aziz showed no interest in book learning, but at seven years of age he was attending all of the daily prayers at the mosque, keeping the Ramadan fast, and quoting verses from the Quran.

He was tall, slender, and muscular like the males of his mother's side. His father, Abdur Rahman, was short and heavy set. Abdur Rahman was the Imam, the religious leader, of the Wahabis.

The Wahabis were serious men, devout and strict, who allowed no luxuries or comforts. Their houses were simply furnished and they forbade singing, music and laughter. These things could distract one's mind from Allah the Great, the Beneficent and Merciful. Their God was kind to those who served Him, but hard and unforgiving to the infidel. It was the duty of the Wahabis to make all men His servants, even by the sword.

Abdul Aziz was taught by his father to walk barefoot on hot stones in the summer months, and was taken on long journeys on horseback. He learned the use of sword and rifle and became agile with horses, mounting, dismounting, and riding without a saddle. Under the guidance of his father, he went without food, water and sleep for periods of time to develop endurance.

Every morning, from the time Abdul Aziz could walk, Abdur Rahman came for him two hours before dawn. They walked together while Abdur Rahman instructed his son in the ways of the Wahabi.

To practice their faith, Muslims must accept the five primary obligations which Islam imposes. Called the Five Pillars of Islam, they are: the profession of faith (*shahadah*), devotional worship or prayer (*salah*), the giving of alms (*zakah*), fasting (*sawm*), and the pilgrimage to Mecca (*hajj*).

Abdur Rahman also taught his son the history of their nation.

"Hundreds of years before Islam came to the Arabs, there was chaos," he said. "The Bedou roamed the desert, attacking each other and anyone else who came into the country. They were pagans."

He told Abdul Aziz how, in 630 AD, the Prophet Mohammed had brought Islam, and with it, unity and control. But it was only a hundred years before the people returned to their tribal ways, and for a thousand years after that nothing changed.

People in the central Arabian province of Nejd warred against each other and against anybody else who ventured into the area. They also began to worship gods of stone and many other things.

Then came Mohammed Ibn Abdul Wahab, in 1750 AD. He preached true Islam, tore off the heresies around the religion and called on all to serve the One True God. He settled under the protection of Mohamed Ibn Saud, ruler of Riyadh.

Ibn Saud made a deal with Abdul Wahab. He provided the force and Abdul Wahab the preaching, and by persuasion or force the Arab nation was united in Islam. The converts were called "Wahabis".

Mohamed Ibn Saud became known as "Saud the Great". After him came another ruler, then another. Sixty years after they began, the Wahabis were raiding as far as Syria and Turkey.

The Turks became angry. They stormed into Arabia, conquered the Nejd and took the then Wahabi ruler, the Saud prince Abdullah, to Constantinople. They executed him in 1818 AD—cutting off his head in front of the Mosque of Santa Sophia in the Great Square. The Wahabis were broken and the tribes once more split up. They began to fight each other again.

"We are of the House of Saud. We are the descendants of Saud the Great," said Abdur Rahman to his son. "Now there is one purpose in my heart—to re-establish his Empire. If only the Arabs could be unified as one nation of devout Wahabis, I could die in peace."

He showed Abdul Aziz a sword, the finest the boy had ever seen. The blade was of Damascus steel, the handle covered with gold and the scabbard inlaid with silver.

"This sword once belonged to Saud the Great," Abdur Rahman said. "One day it will belong again to the Ruler of Arabia."

Abdul Aziz felt safe in the town of Riyadh. The Garden City was a fort with high walls, and its sentries were constantly on guard. All persons wishing to enter had to report for questioning at the gates. At prayer times the gates were locked. Beyond the city stretched the desert, out of which emerged caravans that had dared to brave the raiding Bedou.

The caravans brought goods from other nations around the peninsula and beyond, and Abdul Aziz listened to their gossip and news. The Shammar tribes to the north had united under Mohamad Ibn Rashid, who had made his capital in Hail. Rashid's aim was to take control of Riyadh, for Riyadh was the heart of the Nejd and the Nejd was the heart of Arabia.

Abdul Aziz learned that within Riyadh there were factions. His father was one of four brothers— the other three being Abdullah, Saud and Mohamed. For several years, Abdullah, Mohamed, and Saud and his sons fought amongst each other to gain supremacy in Riyadh. Then there was murder in the streets, and even in the palace, as the people of Riyadh took sides.

One by one, Abdur Rahman's brothers died or were killed in battle and finally, Rashid's warriors from the north invaded and took over the city. Now Abdur Rahman was the only one of his siblings left.

Rashid decided to put a governor in charge of Riyadh—Salim, a sheik of Shammar, but left Abdur Rahman in the palace because he was a peaceable man, and had influence with the Wahabis.

However, Abdur Rahman could not stand by and see Riyadh ruled by Rashid. He tried to enlist the help of the sons of his brother Saud, to wrest control of Riyadh back from the Rashid men, but his nephews insisted that they alone had the right to leadership.

Secretly, he tried to get the people behind him, planning attacks from within and outside the town, but the people were afraid. Rashid had a strong presence. Once before the people had rioted and many of them had been hanged by Salim.

Abdur Rahman was in danger, surrounded by spies and traitors including his own nephews. Salim, the Governor, finally discovered Abdur Rahman's subversive activities and decided to do away with him.

On the last day of the great festival of Eid in 1891, Salim organized to pay Abdur Rahman a formal visit. After the customary greetings, he would ask that all the males in the family be gathered for an important message. When all were present, Salim would order his guards to kill them.

Abdur Rahman learned of the plan and decided to counter with a trick of his own. He armed the men he had, and kept them at the ready. He met Salim and his guards with just a few of the family present, including ten-year-old Abdul Aziz and his personal slave.

Greetings and congratulations were exchanged, courtesies extended, coffee drunk and trifles spoken of. Then Salim asked for all the males of the family to be summoned.

Abdur Rahman motioned to a slave, with the pre-arranged signal, and suddenly there was pandemonium as his men swarmed into the room.

Abdul Aziz was protected by the strong arm of his huge slave, but he found a peephole under that arm. He watched as his father's men overwhelmed and slaughtered the Rashid guards and dragged Salim away.

Fired up by the victory, the townspeople rallied and drove out the remainder of Rashid's forces. For weeks Abdur Rahman and Rashid's men raided against each other. Finally Abdur Rahman was confined to Riyadh, with the countryside around the township under control of the Rashid. Food and water dwindled. Rashid's warriors cut down the palms around the city, destroyed irrigation channels and ruined the gardens.

The townspeople had had enough. They demanded that Abdur Rahman make peace with the Rashid and threatened to rise against him when he refused. He reluctantly sent out a truce party, with young Abdul Aziz along as surety.

The Rashid were tired and ready to make a bargain. Salim was handed over to them, and they agreed to leave Abdur Rahman in charge as their governor in Riyadh.

However, as the Rashid began their journey north, the people began to chase them. Abdur Rahman joined in. Young Abdul Aziz rode along on a camel with his black slave, following the fighting men as they sallied forth.

The Rashid turned and lashed out, smashing their way back to the city. Abdur Rahman could not sustain the fight. Grabbing Abdul Aziz and thrusting him into a saddle bag on his own camel, he turned and raced for the city walls.

"Salim was right," the Rashid shouted, "the Sauds are full of treachery! This time we will wipe them out completely."

They took up positions outside the walls and waited for reinforcements.

The townspeople were afraid to support Abdur Rahman again. They did not want another siege. At dead of night, Abdur Rahman received reports that the Rashid's reinforcements were on their way and would be at the city within hours. His slaves loaded all that they could onto the camels, and then the family of Abdul Rahman swiftly passed through the eastern gate of Riyadh.

Abdul Aziz and his brother Mohamed rode one camel. They passed through palm groves and then the Dahna Desert, and finally into the Hasa, in the south east of Arabia.

There Abdur Rahman found Hithlain, the Sheik of the Ajman tribes, and claimed sanctuary. Hithlain was bound by the code of desert courtesy to give it to him but was sullen all the same. Abdur Rahman's nephews were amongst the Ajman, and demanded that their uncle be thrown out. Rashid also ordered Hithlain to give him up.

Abdur Rahman was apprehensive. He feared that the treacherous Ajman would turn on him. Abdul Aziz became ill with rheumatic fever at this time, so

Abdur Rahman sent him and the rest of his family to Bahrain, the island of pearl fishers, off the east coast of Arabia.

Alone now, Abdur Rahman tried to muster support to retake Riyadh. He gathered a few Bedou who were ready for raiding, and they made towards Riyadh. The people of the Nejd were no help, and the Rashid garrison drove them off. Discouraged, Abdur Rahman returned to Hasa.

The Turkish governor of the region sent for him on his arrival. The Turks thought themselves the lords of Arabia. However they only held the fringes— Yemen, Asir, Hejaz, Kuwait and Hasa. In the desert they had no real power and depended on tribal rivalries to retain some control. They were afraid of the strength of Rashid and offered Abdur Rahman assistance to take and rule the Nejd, on condition that he acknowledge Turkish sovereignty and pay tribute.

Abdur Rahman refused at once. He was an Arab and a Wahabi! He would not bow to the Turks! They were intruders and infidels; he would not allow them to interfere. The Turks threatened him, accusing him of being a dangerous man and leading revolts against them in conjunction with the Sheik of Qatar.

Now Abdur Rahman was truly a refugee. He took Abdul Aziz, who had now recovered from his illness, his younger son Mohamed, and the boys' cousin, Jiluwi, south through Jabrin to the Rub Al Khali, the Empty Quarter. By the wells of Khiran, he found the Murra tribesmen grazing camels in the scrub and claimed protection from them.

For many months the Sauds lived among the Murra. These were the most primitive tribes in Arabia, long-haired, lean men with wild eyes and crafty spirits. They lived on dates kept from the last season, camel milk, and occasionally meat from hare, gazelle or deer. The water from the wells was too salty to drink.

They also ate *jabru* (rats which lived amongst the rocks), *dhub* lizards and ostrich eggs. A luxury the Murra sometimes enjoyed was liver of camel rubbed in salt. Not fit things for a Moslem to eat, Abdur Rahman complained.

The Murra were true Bedou, continually wandering in search of fodder for animals. They were fierce in their raids, attacking without warning, killing and plundering then vanishing back into the mighty desert, where none could follow. They raided to the Hadramaut and Oman, stealing prized camels.

Abdul Aziz threw himself completely into the life of the Bedou. He lived under the stars, traveling with the Murra, raiding and hunting, learning the ways of the desert. He learned how to track footprints, interpret signs in the sand, how to make long journeys by camel, and how to live on slim rations of dates and camel milk. He became lean, wiry and ready for action.

But his father despised the life. He thought the Murra were pagans, worse than infidels, and his pride suffered by having to live with them. Their raids into northern territories had no effect on the powerful Rashid and Abdur Rahman despaired of ever achieving his ambition. He was over fifty now and wanted the comfort of his wife and children around him.

He tried repeatedly to gain protection from any of the Sheiks, but nobody wanted to risk helping him as he had many enemies. At last, to his delight,

Mohamed, the Sheik of Kuwait, sent an invitation, offering him a monthly allowance while he was with them. Abdur Rahman collected the rest of his family from Bahrain and settled down in Kuwait. It was now 1890.

Kuwait was a dry yellow town of bricks and twisting alleys, along the shore of the Persian Gulf. There was a sandy beach, and a shallow harbor with a basic breakwater. The red sands shimmered out from the town in a haze of heat. A few small tamarisk trees provided limited shade.

The family crowded into the three rooms of a small house which opened onto a courtyard. It was a poor hovel by comparison to the palace in Riyadh. A narrow alley ran from the house down to the shore, where shipwrights and sail makers worked. Pearl fishers hauled up and serviced their boats here. The beach was filthy, and stank under the sun and flies.

Abdul Aziz was curious enough to wander here often, and made friends among the pearlers and merchants. He sat by the open cafés, listened to talk of seamen and desert sheiks, and played knucklebones with other youths. He quarreled and fought with them, held hands with his friends as young Arabs do, and played jokes on shopkeepers until they chased him away.

Kuwait was the gateway between the north and the Gulf, a crossroads where people mingled—people from India, Persia, Syria, Armenia, and all over the Middle East. Goods came in on ships and left on caravans bound for central Arabia and for Syria.

Abdul Aziz joined his father for prayers five times a day, and observed the Ramadan fast when it came around. He was big for his age, strong and tough from his months with the desert Bedou, and outgoing.

The Sheik was friendly, but not generous. He rarely paid the allowance he had promised to Abdur Rahman. The Turks now realized the full strength of Rashid and his tribes, and wanted to use Abdur Rahman against them. Again they offered to allow him back to Riyadh as their figurehead. He refused angrily.

Now the Turks declared that they would stop his allowance altogether—and so Abdur Rahman discovered that it was the Turkish Governor in Hasa who had secretly arranged for Mohamed of Kuwait to invite Abdur Rahman and his family to stay there. It was the *Turks* who had been supporting him, who had guaranteed Mohamed an allowance to keep his guests!

Abdur Rahman was furious at the trick. He would have paid back the money if he could, but he had nothing left of his own and often had to borrow to feed his family.

Abdul Aziz was now fifteen. His mother discussed marriage—she would find a Bedou girl for him to marry, to keep him pure and his thoughts from wandering. The wedding day approached, but there was no money for celebrations so the marriage was postponed. Then one of Abdul Aziz's rich merchant friends from the waterfront offered to pay for the wedding.

The poor young Bedou girl only lived for six months. Abdul Aziz was not even sure that he had loved her. He married again and had a son, Turki, within the year.

Mohamed, the Sheik of Kuwait, had a brother, Mubarak, but the two of them did not get along. Mubarak paid visits to Abdur Rahman from time to time. He spent all he owned in gambling and fine living, sold his mother's jewels to pay debts, and became penniless.

"Mohamed hates me," Mubarak said. "The people of the town like me, so he is afraid of me. He keeps me poor and tries to make me look foolish whenever he can."

One day, when Abdul Aziz was seventeen years old, Mubarak whispered to him, "Things are about to change. Watch and see!"

That night Mubarak, with a cousin and a servant, stole into the palace and murdered his brother. Then he pronounced himself Sheik of Kuwait, and the people celebrated.

Two weeks later a visitor came to Abdur Rahman's house.

"Mohamed Al Rashid is dead," he said. "His son, Abdul Aziz Ibn Rashid, is no more than a common raider, with no strength of character and no control of his people. The people of Nejd are ready for a change. The time is ripe for a take-over!"

Abdul Aziz went to his father.

"I want to go," he said. "I must go! How can we sit here in this foreign country and not try to win back our heritage? Here we are, wasting away in poverty."

Abdur Rahman looked tired and discouraged.

"I can't go with you," he said. "I have no men, no substance and no enthusiasm. You are young. If you go, take my blessing with you—that's all I have to give."

So Abdul Aziz went to see Mubarak.

"Sorry, I can't help you," said Mubarak. "The Rashid would give me trouble. If you go, you go alone—I can't be seen to help you. I wish you well."

Abdul Aziz borrowed an old, mangy camel and set off with a few friends. The young men traveled at night so they wouldn't be seen. They made some raids for supplies and were encouraged by their success.

Close to Riyadh, they entered a village and discovered the awful truth—the people were not ready to revolt, and would not support Abdul Aziz. He set off again, but his camel stumbled and fell and would not rise again.

"I'm finished," he said. "Let's go back to Kuwait. Although we're poor, we are safe there."

The men began walking, and then hitched a ride with a caravan. They arrived in Kuwait in disgrace, tired and discouraged. Abdul Aziz's sister Nura, who was just as ambitious and daring as he, sympathized with his failure and urged him not to give up.

Mubarak liked Abdul Aziz. He invited the young man to his house often over the next two years and taught him worldly wisdom. The year Mubarak came to power, he had received consuls from England, Germany and Russia, and had listened to them and their offers. With the power and responsibility of governing Kuwait, he had changed from a frivolous spendthrift to a shrewd and careful ruler.

Mubarak included Abdur Rahman and Abdul Aziz in his conferences. However, Abdur Rahman disapproved of Mubarak's past life. By Wahabi standards, Mubarak was immoral and lax in his religion. He lived in style and luxury, was irregular about prayers, and the ceilings in his house bore pictures of naked girls. Mubarak also smoked tobacco and was entertained by dancing girls.

Soon, Abdur Rahman refused to visit Mubarak in the palace and forbade Abdul Aziz to do so. However Abdul Aziz continued to visit in secret, and developed a strong friendship with Mubarak.

Abdul Aziz sat in on audiences with people from all over Europe. The young man learned much about the outside world and how to govern. He saw how Mubarak handled people, and how problems of other countries could affect Kuwait. He became aware of new ideas and customs, including many things which were forbidden or unknown in Riyadh.

Kuwait itself was difficult to rule. Its population had come from many parts of Arabia. Cheating, brawling, theft, and murder were common, and Mubarak dealt swiftly and firmly with offenders. The town prospered and its inhabitants felt secure.

Abdul Aziz learned quickly. He was usually good natured and friendly and, although he was a Wahabi, he was quick to laughter. He boasted to his companions of how he was heir to Riyadh and Nejd, and would one day evict Rashid and rule the whole of Arabia. They laughed at him, reminding him of his failed attempt on Riyadh and the collapse of his mangy camel. This angered him.

World events began to affect Kuwait. The Kaiser of Germany wanted to expand his boundaries, and looked to the East and India. The Kaiser allied with the Sultan of Turkey and proclaimed himself friend and protector of the Arabs. Germany began to press down through the East, but England held all the roads, with the exception of that from Turkey through the Arab countries into the Persian Gulf.

So Germany planned a railway from Constantinople through Baghdad to Kuwait—the gateway to the Gulf. For a hundred years the English from India had been pressing into the Middle East, making allies with the Gulf countries and gaining control. They were determined that Germany would not establish itself here.

Mubarak saw that the English would be allies but would not aim to take over his country. The Germans, on the other hand, would swallow up Kuwait if they established their railway. He played for time, postponing a decision, until word came from his spies that the Germans had approached the Turks and had urged that they depose Mubarak. Immediately he called the English and signed an agreement with them.

He was just in time—the Turks had decided to stir up Rashid against Mubarak, saying that whoever ruled central Arabia could have Kuwait. Turkey would support Rashid with arms and finance. They also pointed out that Kuwait was sheltering their old enemy—the Saud family. Rashid agreed at once to attack!

Mubarak saw the danger. He had no fighting men, and knew that he must find allies. He sent messengers to find tribes who would side with him against Rashid—the Murra, Ajman, Mutair, and Muntafik.

Mubarak decided to attack Rashid, catching the troops unprepared, and called on allies from around Arabia. He marched out with ten thousand men, including Abdur Rahman, and sent Abdul Aziz south to harry Riyadh.

Abdul Aziz was eager for action. He asked Jiluwi, his cousin, to go with him, and also some men of Nejd who were in Kuwait. They traveled swiftly through the desert and found the people of Nejd ready to join them. Soon Abdul Aziz had a large force, and swept toward Riyadh.

But Mubarak, in the north, had been failed by his allies when he met the first wave of Rashid men. He had been defeated, and was retreating towards Kuwait. Abdul Aziz's forces disbanded when they heard of it, and fled. Abdul Aziz rushed back to Kuwait, with Rashid troops smashing the villages of Nejd as they followed him.

As Rashid warriors approached Kuwait, Mubarak was in a panic. He did not have the troops or the supplies to resist. Yet again Abdur Rahman was about to flee for his life with his family, when the English came to the rescue. They warned off the Rashid men, and sent a cruiser to reinforce their position. The Rashid melted back into the desert.

Although defeated by Rashid, Abdul Aziz refused to give in. At twenty he was tough and determined, ready for war. Tall and muscular, he also had a strong and persuasive personality. Now he was furious. He cursed the Ajman and other deserters, and the Rashid for murdering his people in the Nejd.

Again he went to Mubarak. He blamed Mubarak for poor planning, and urged him, unsuccessfully, to try again. Other sheiks refused to help—they would not stand up to the Rashid.

Abdur Rahman tried to discourage his son, saying the time was not right, that he should try again later, but Abdul Aziz would not listen. He would not hide any longer; he was tired of six years of sitting around, talking. It was no life for a man of the desert, especially a man of the house of Saud. He wanted to fight!

"Give me a camel or a horse and let me go," he said. "By Allah I will win, and if not, I will die in battle."

Weeks went by and Abdul Aziz kept on at Mubarak. Finally Mubarak gave him thirty camels, thirty rifles, ammunition, and two hundred riyals of gold.

"Do what you can to the Rashid," he told Abdul Aziz, " but if they cause me trouble I will deny that I ever assisted you."

Abdul Aziz then went to his father and arranged for his wife and his son to remain in his household. He found thirty friends who were eager to go with him, including Jiluwi, his cousin, and his brother Mohamed.

His mother tearfully tried to dissuade him, sure that he would die or be doomed to fail again. On the other hand, his sister Nura urged him on and Abdur Rahman gave him a blessing.

It was late summer and very hot. One dark night Abdul Aziz and his companions slipped away without further ado, beyond the city to where their camels were waiting.

They moved with speed, as Abdul Aziz had learned from the Murra, and did not weigh themselves down with food or equipment. He encouraged his men to ration their food and only took enough dates and dried curds for a week. They made sure that their tracks were not easy to follow; they camped in hollows, and used sentries at night. They made swift approaches to villages, looting them and then dashing away.

Abdul Aziz slept only a little, an hour or two at a time. No man dared to face him; he was an inspiration to his men with his courage and energy. "See how he fights!" they marveled. Speedily he went, scattering the enemy.

First he moved toward Hasa, attacked Ajman and Rashid there and made off with loot. He rallied the Bedou and hounded the Rashid across the country. He tried to rouse the people of Nejd and Riyadh to stand against the Rashid once more, but they would not cooperate.

Then began the difficulties. Raids began to fail, money became scarce, and their camels were in poor condition. Some of the beasts had been mangy to begin with. The Bedou deserted him and the Rashid began to harry him. He was chased from Hasa by the Ajman and the Turks. Curse them—by Allah he would see the last of them or die trying.

Then he turned south towards the Rub Al Khali, where a messenger from Kuwait caught up with him.

"Mubarak and your father are anxious about you. Advise you to return to Kuwait. The time is not yet for action."

Abdul Aziz thought carefully. Things were going wrong, yet his belief was strong.

"Come with me," he said to the messenger, and called his men together.

Amongst the few palms at Jabrin, Abdul Aziz talked frankly to his men. He was determined to go on. Who would go with him? Some left. Fifty remained, along with their slaves, including the original thirty from Kuwait. Abdul Aziz asked them to swear an oath to stand by him.

"Go back," he said to the messenger. "Tell my father what you have seen and heard. Tell him that I will no longer wait patiently, while our country is under the heel of the Rashid. I will not come back until I have succeeded. All things are in the hands of Allah the Most Merciful."

Abdul Aziz thought carefully. Raids would accomplish little. He must plan a dramatic take-over. He would aim for Riyadh itself! One of his men went in to spy and returned with a report.

"There is a strong Rashid garrison in the town, holding the Almasmak fort. The Governor, Ajlan, lives in a house opposite the fort. The people of Riyadh and the Nejd are unhappy—they hate the Rashid, but they are afraid. They are praying for a Saud to return and rule, but they will never rise alone. There must be a leader."

Abdul Aziz realized that he must use cunning; he did not have the numbers to attack openly. He sent out rumors that all his men had deserted. Then he made for the Rub Al Khali, and waited there for fifty days. His men were sorely tested. They were men of action and could not bear to wait idly, although they trusted their leader.

It needed all of Abdul Aziz's powers of persuasion to maintain that loyalty—he argued, threatened, appealed to their pride, and held them to his purpose. They had few rations, and only seldom ate meat, when they could kill a sand-deer. They stole water from wells, taking care to cover their tracks.

Now the month of fasting began. Many of them kept the fast rigidly, including Abdul Aziz and Jiluwi. They took nothing to eat or drink from an hour before sunrise until sunset, every day.

On the twentieth day of Ramadan, after the breaking of the fast and the evening prayer, Abdul Aziz decided to move. The small band traveled carefully through the nights, hiding by day. There was no moon, so sentries moved ahead to prevent the men from stumbling into encampments and giving themselves away. The camels were in bad shape, many with mange and very lean.

At the wells of Abu Jifan they celebrated the Id Al Fitr, the festival ending the fast, and reached the Tuwaiq hills close to Riyadh. Now they must move quickly; there were villages—they might be seen, they must reach Riyadh before a warning could be sent.

The camels were forced to speed up. Finally the small band reached the Groves of Dil Ashuaib, an hour and a half's walk from Riyadh. Abdul Aziz selected some of the men to go with him and left the rest with the animals, with orders to come only if he sent for them. If they heard nothing for more than twenty-four hours they should go to Kuwait and tell his father that he was either dead or a prisoner of the Rashid.

On foot, he and forty men crept through the palm groves that separated them from the town. When they arrived at Shamsieh, the palm groves ended. The convoy stopped. Abdul Aziz cut down a palm tree. He chose Jiluwi and six others, leaving the rest of the men with his brother Mohamed to await orders.

"If no message comes to you by tomorrow, go home, for you know that we are dead. There is no power or might save in Allah."

Abdul Aziz and his small party of men stole through the gardens in darkness, carrying the palm trunk. They followed a twisted path over mud walls and across irrigation channels, listening for sounds of an alarm.

Finally they came close to the town wall, near the great cemetery where the road to Mecca runs, and crouched in the dry moat. As they listened, they could hear sentries in the fort above. The watchman cried out on his rounds and moved on. Then there was silence. They had not been seen.

Abdul Aziz put the palm trunk against the wall, and one by one he and his men crept up it and dropped into the street. It was now mid January. The night air was winter-crisp, and everyone was indoors.

The young warriors made their way carefully down the street, following Abdul Aziz. He led them to the house of Jowaisir, a cowherd who lived close to the house of the Governor.

He knocked at the door, and a woman called out to enquire who it was.

"I am from the Governor—I come to see about buying two cows," he said.

"Go away! Do you think we are harlots? Go away. This is no time to come knocking on doors where there are decent women," she cried.

"If you do not open, I will tell the Governor tomorrow, and Jowaisir will suffer!"

A few minutes later the door opened a crack and a man looked out. The light of the room speared out from behind him. Two of Abdul Aziz's men grabbed the man and held his mouth, while the others pressed through the door and closed it behind them. The man was an old servant from the palace and was overjoyed to see Abdul Aziz.

"It is the master!" he cried, and called his family to welcome the young man. He gave them the information they needed. "The fort is full of Rashid soldiers. They don't take any special care, and do not seem to expect attack. The Governor usually sleeps in the fort. Just after dawn his horse is brought to him and he either rides or walks over to his house. He always has guards around him. His home is two doors away from here, and there are no sentries."

Abdul Aziz and his men crept up to the rooftop, and moved like shadows to the next house. Here they found a man and his wife, asleep in bed. They wrapped them in their bedclothes and tied them up securely.

The Governor's house was joined to this one but stood a level higher. Abdul Aziz and his men had to climb on each others' shoulders to reach the roof top and there they lay panting. Once again they had not been discovered. On bare feet they crept down the stairs, found the servants in the basement and locked them in a room together, under guard. On the second floor they found the Governor's bedroom.

"Stay here at the door," Abdul Aziz ordered his men. "Only Jiluwi and I will go in."

Jiluwi carried a lighted candle, which he shielded with one hand. Abdul Aziz slid a cartridge into his rifle. There were two women in the bed. One of them sat up and shrieked in terror. Abdul Aziz threw his hand across her mouth. Jiluwi wrestled with the other woman.

"Do not make a sound or I will kill you!" said Abdul Aziz. As the candle light reached her face, he recognized her. Her father had worked for his father in the palace.

"Mutlib!" he exclaimed. "What are you doing here?"

"I married the Governor," she said insolently. "What of it?"

"Slut!" said Abdul Aziz disdainfully.

"My lord, I am no slut. I only married after you left us. Why do you come here?"

"I have come to kill Ajlan," said Abdul Aziz simply.

"Ajlan is in the fort. He has over eighty men with him. You should escape while he is still asleep, or he will find you and kill you."

"When does he return to the house?" asked Abdul Aziz.

"After the sun is an hour into the sky."

"Then stay quiet, for if you make a sound we will cut your throats."

The men locked the two women in with the servants and began another vigil, four hours before dawn. In the front of the house was a large room.

"See here," said Jiluwi. "We have a good view of the fort from the windows!"

The fort had a double iron-studded door in a high wall. On top of the wall, a sentry walked his beat.

"Let's take the Governor when he comes out, then we'll go into the fort," said Abdul Aziz. "Send two men to get Mohamed and the others."

They set watch on the windows, and recited from the Quran. They prayed, and made peace with those they had argued with. Some slept a little. Their reinforcements arrived with the morning and they refreshed themselves with coffee, dates and bread. Then it was time for morning prayers. Abdul Aziz performed the duties of Imam, bowing deeply towards Mecca.

When sunlight stained the wall of the fort opposite, there was movement. The horses were being led towards the fort.

"Four of you stand by the windows," ordered Abdul Aziz. "Have your rifles ready. As soon as you see us running across the square, fire on the guards! The rest of you, follow me."

The iron studded doors opened wide, and Ajlan, the governor, came out to the horses, his guards behind him.

"Now!" muttered Abdul Aziz and ran towards Ajlan with a great shout.

Ajlan spun around, startled, and grabbed for his sword. Abdul Aziz held the sword back with his rifle and the two men fell, wrestling, to the ground.

The Governor's guards fled to the fort. One hit out at Jiluwi, who felled him with his sword. Ajlan struggled desperately. He broke free and ran for the gate of the fort, shouting for assistance. Abdul Aziz fired at him, striking his arm, making him release his sword, and then dived for his legs as he grabbed a post.

Soldiers rushed from within the fort as Abdul Aziz and his men swarmed towards it, and all was noise and confusion as they writhed together on the steps. Above the courtyard guards fired, and tumbled blocks of stone down. Ajlan wrested a leg free and kicked Abdul Aziz in the groin, causing him to release his grip.

A guard tried to drag the Governor through the gate and close it, but Jiluwi and three others threw themselves at the gate. Then firing came from all the walls of the garrison. Ajlan ran across the courtyard towards the mosque, with Abdul Aziz and Jiluwi after him. As they reached the steps, Jiluwi swung his sword mightily and Ajlan fell beneath it.

Abdul Aziz and his band were seriously outnumbered, but they smelled victory and together they surged back up the staircase and into the fort.

Half the garrison were dead or wounded when the onslaught ended, and the rest were surrounded in one room.

A shout went up from the city walls, and the people of Riyadh rallied. They rose up, and wiped out the remaining Rashid in the city.

Back in Kuwait, Abdur Rahman received a messenger. The family was summoned immediately. Abdur Rahman was moist-eyed, but wore a new look of pride and resolve on his face.

"My son Abdul Aziz has conquered the Rashid. The Sauds rule again in Riyadh!"

Abdur Rahman made his way to Riyadh, where Abdul Aziz met him in delight and hailed him as the new king.

A few days later, the old man called a meeting with the *Ulema*, the religious council, and the elders of the tribes.

"I have always been a man of action and ready to fight," he announced, "but now Riyadh needs a young man to lead. I am growing old, and no longer want to be a leader. I wish to pass rulership on to my son, although I am willing to encourage and advise."

Then he called Abdul Aziz to him.

"Take this, my son. It belonged to Saud the Great, a hundred years ago. Now it is yours."

The people gasped as Abdur Rahman brought forth the magnificent sword and placed it in Abdul Aziz's hand. It belonged to the ruler of Riyadh, of Nejd, and of all Arabia. Abdul Aziz would live to be worthy of it.

It was 1902 when Abdul Aziz Ibn Saud captured Riyadh. He gained final control of the Nejd in 1912 and became king of the Hejaz in 1926. By 1932 he had gained control of most of the Arab peninsula and established the Kingdom of Saudi Arabia.

Acknowledgements: "Lord of Arabia" by H.C. Armstrong. Published by Penguin, 1938

12 - FRIENDS AND ACQUAINTANCES

GERRY AND JACKIE Donovan were two of the most likeable people I had ever met. They were always smiling and had a fresh, carefree attitude to life that was enviable. They also had a whacky sense of humor. Once when their daughter arrived at Dhahran airport, Gerry went to meet her with a pig mask on. Another time he held up a placard with her name on it.

Gerry and Jackie had been in RT for so long that they were part of the establishment. One of the rooms in their large, sprawling mansion was dedicated to cats and kittens, and the rest of the house was full of antiques and zany items they had picked up from around the world. Their other great love was the theater and Gerry directed and produced numerous plays with the Ras Tanura Players' Group, as well as taking active roles onstage in many of them.

Some of the best parties were at Gerry and Jackie's house. The 'Helga' parties continued for several years, with skits, prizes, and great food. The three 'Sheiks'—Sheik Rattle and Roll, Sheik 'n' Bake and Sheik Al Eg attended at least one of them.

One day, Gerry told us, he had just driven through the gate on his way to Rahima when he remembered something he should have taken with him. He spun around and went back inside the compound. The guard, probably seeking something to brighten his dull life, stopped him and demanded to see his ID card. It irked Gerry.

"You know me!" he said. "I've only just come out—I forgot something. Don't tell me I have to get my card out."

The guard was unyielding and Gerry's bent for drama came to the fore.

"OK," he said. "I'll get my ID. Just wait a minute."

He struggled with his wallet and out came the driver's license.

"Oops! That's not it," he said.

He struggled some more. Out came some receipts.

"Nope," he said. "It has to be here somewhere." Behind him, several car engines revved.

"Never mind then, just go!" The guard gestured impatiently.

"No, no. You asked for my ID and I will get it for you. Ahhh, here it is," Gerry said at last, flicking the ID card out of his wallet and out the window. He leaped out of the door and flung himself under the car after it, while horns began to sound. Cars were now backed up behind him to the highway.

"Here—I have it!" He waved the card triumphantly in the air.

"Go! Go! Just go!" said the guard, who by now was frantic to be rid of him.

Sarah and Hugh Stanley were friends who lived on the beachfront in RT. I warmed to Sarah's helpful, friendly nature, while Hugh's dry humor kept everyone chuckling.

Hugh had to have rehabilitation for two serious injuries while in Saudi Arabia. Both were sustained while driving quad cars, or ATV's, out on desert dunes. Fortunately other campers were able to rescue him on both occasions and get him to hospital.

On the first occasion he had broken his shoulder in two places. As he waited in agony in the hospital foyer the police were called, as it had technically been a 'motor vehicle accident.'

In Saudi Arabia, an accident involving a motor vehicle is a very serious incident, and must be fully investigated in case anybody is at fault and stands to be punished. Even if there are no injuries it could be several hours before the persons involved are cleared, and in some cases a driver may end up in jail for weeks until the cause of the accident is settled to the satisfaction of the police. Blame may be apportioned to more than one individual.

In Hugh's case, it was several hours before he could gain medical attention for his fractures. Finally, after many forms had been completed, he was released for treatment. The shoulder was pinned and it was months before he gained maximum function in his arm.

The second time Hugh fell from the quad he suffered a compound fracture of his lower leg. I visited him after the bone had been pinned in surgery and he was recuperating at home.

"What happened?" I asked, expecting a repeat of the previous scenario.

Hugh looked at me with a straight face.

"Well," he said in his Texan drawl, "I have almost finished writing a three page report for the company. I'll read it to you."

He began a long account of a stroll in the desert and over dunes, ending with a dramatic fall including a roll down a steep hill and an entrapment of his affected limb in a hole. By the time he finished tears of laughter were running down my face.

"Well that's my story," said Hugh, with the hint of a twinkle in his eye. "And I almost believe it myself."

David and Jenny Campbell were two of the longest-serving Aramcons I knew. David was a gentle giant, a special teacher, and Jenny worked as a welcome lady for Ras Tanura new hires. David and Jenny enjoyed a weekend in Bahrain as much as any of us.

On one of these excursions Jenny needed to use the bathroom in the middle of the night. Stark naked and somewhat disoriented, she suddenly found herself in the hallway outside her hotel room. And suddenly the door slipped out of her grasp and closed with a gentle click behind her!

What to do? Should she bang on the door to wake up her husband and risk someone else opening their door to see what the commotion was? Terrified, she knocked gently on the door and after several minutes David woke up. He went to the door, put his eye to the peephole, and realized that another, very worried eye was looking back at him! She was a very relieved lady to get back inside that door without waking anybody else in the establishment.

Early in the days of company operations, the residential compounds had more freedoms. In these little Western oases, expatriates enjoyed most of the privileges they had in their home countries. The Aramco compounds sported the first and only movie theaters in Kingdom, pork stores, organized dances, religious services and open-air Christmas pageants.

Alcohol was also sold in the early days. It was commonly known as *'siddiqi'* or just plain *'sid'*. The word meant 'my friend' in Arabic and was considered an appropriate term for moonshine.

The company gave stills to the expatriate employees at one time, so they could make alcohol for their own use at home. Special ground-floor rooms attached to the garages were designed for the purpose, with water taps, drains, and two hundred and forty volt power supply.

Long before I arrived stills had become illegal, but Security tended to turn a blind eye to them, unless employees were caught profiteering from them.

Running a still required care and attention. Dangerous vapors collected under some circumstances, and any spark, such as formed when turning electric appliances or a light switch off, could trigger an explosion.

Those who became careless in their operations faced real danger. Windows shattered, house fires started and people were severely burned in several instances during my employment with the company. Whenever a still exploded, the official explanation would invariably implicate a faulty oven or air-conditioning unit and the offending employee would be quietly shipped home.

A friend, Jack, owned a still which he monitored with an adjustable temperature alarm. Once a year he would carefully process five gallons of pure alcohol which could subsequently be diluted to make alcoholic drinks of an acceptable standard. On occasion he would give it away, but usually kept it for his own use and for his Christmas party, which was a major event on the compound. His hooch, which was of an unusually high quality, was highly prized by his guests.

On Jack's departure from Kingdom he lent the still to Greg, a fellow countryman, on condition that he had it shipped out with his belongings when he retired from Aramco.

The deal sat sweetly with Greg, who began to process rough moonshine for sale on camp. He didn't bother with the temperature alarm, which Jack had so carefully installed. One night he left the still running while he and the family went to bed. During the night, his wife was woken up by a strange odor. She shook Greg awake, and he went downstairs to investigate while she got the children out of bed from the room above the still.

The story goes that Greg passed out from the fumes, falling against the wall and knocking the light switch off as he fell. The spark caused an explosion which burnt him severely but which probably saved him from dying in the fumes. His wife and children, fortunately, were safe. Greg spent three months in hospital recuperating from his burns, before his employment was terminated without benefits.

Another man on camp was blown out of his patio when his still exploded. He cut his feet on glass as he dragged the incriminating evidence out of the house and down to the beach, throwing it into the bay. Unfortunately for him, as the tide went out it revealed the still, high and dry!

13 - WEEKEND ESCAPES

"DO YOU EVER go to Bahrain?" the young Saudi Arab asked.

"Not much," I replied. "I've been there a couple of times and it was OK but I'd rather go camping here in Kingdom."

A mischievous smile crept over his face.

"I go to Bahrain every weekend," he said. "I go to Bahrain...to drink...water."

Laughter engulfed us both. Each of us knew that what he drank in Bahrain was not water!

In 1986 the King Fahad Causeway, linking Saudi Arabia to Bahrain, was opened. This amazing sixteen mile long structure across the Gulf of Bahrain had about six checkpoints and took about an hour to get across on a good day. Aramco employees quickly learned the best times to avoid the rush and made the most of the proximity of this liberal island country.

Bahrain is an island of about ten by thirty miles in area with a very long history. It has always been a trading point in the Middle East; from approximately 3200 BC the Dilmun Empire ruled for around 2000 years. Prior to the development of the petroleum industry, Bahrain was the pearling capital of the world, with divers risking their lives free diving to secure a prize specimen. Nowadays, Bahrain is best known for its trading in oil and finance. It is a constitutional monarchy, with a Prime Minister and a cabinet of fifteen to rule the country.

Although it is an Islamic state, there is remarkable religious freedom and tolerance of lifestyle in Bahrain. World-class hotels, restaurants and shopping attract visitors, and alcohol is freely available. It was no secret that Saudi Arabs, as well as westerners, regularly slaked their thirst here.

Within Saudi Aramco, as more and more Saudi Arabs became senior employees and were thus entitled to live in the Western compounds, rules were adjusted to accommodate Islamic ideals. The freedoms that Westerners had been able to enjoy became increasingly restricted. As the local population became more and more comfortable within the compounds, westerners began to feel some deprivation.

Dancing was one of the small pleasures being phased out, and so 1993 saw the last yacht club ball in Ras Tanura. As members moved in and out of the hall and decorated it in black and gold, curious Arabs stood by, watching.

"Is this a wedding?" one asked, finally.

"Yes," someone said. "It's a wedding."

Hence hotels in Bahrain became the venues for end of year festivities for various special groups after that. Bahrain presented a wonderful mixture of eastern and western cultures, where some of the best hotels and restaurants in the world could be found.

Delicious buffets were served here, with tables loaded with delicacies from all over the world. Chefs prepared crepes, omelets and pancakes to order; views through wide windows spanned the island city with views across the causeway and the beautiful waters of the Arabian Gulf.

It is hard to describe the ambience of these wonderful resorts and the abundance of the many delicacies westerners living in the Middle East came to accept as regular fare. Bahrain is said by some to have been the original Garden of Eden; perhaps it really was.

In Bahrain one could buy the latest in fashion, gadgets, oriental carpets, antiques, electronic goods, spectacles, sports shoes and many other items duty-free, at reasonable prices.

Beyond the city sprawled the *suqs*, often known as the old town, with tiny hole-in-the-wall shops, stalls crowded around narrow lanes filled with jostling pedestrians, vendors and the occasional vehicle inching its way through the confusion.

Shoppers hunted for bargains amongst beautiful fabrics, an infinity of spices, Arabic and western clothing, shoes, kitchenware, gold and many other things. Just to wander through the *suqs* could set your blood tingling.

There were other attractions in Bahrain besides food, alcohol and shopping. The Bahrain National Museum was interesting, with an impressive display on the Dilmun Empire.

The Tree of Life was also worth a visit—a flourishing 500 year old acacia tree, which stands alone in a very dry and barren place with no apparent water supply. A legend says that if you touch it you will live longer.

Then there were the mosques: Al-Fateh mosque—the lovely building on the outskirts of the city, and the ruins of the Al-Khamis mosque, which dates from around the eleventh century and has been partially restored.

And there were the forts. Arad Fort, a Portuguese building of mud, stone and straw, was built around the fifteenth century, though not much is known about its beginnings. It dates from the fourteenth century, although excavations show ruins from around 2300 BC. Riffa Fort was built in 1812, with an amazing wind tunnel which is cool on the hottest days.

If you were inclined to go diving, that could also be arranged. Pearl divers have been operating in the waters here for a thousand years and more. There are colorful fish and corals, and old wrecks to explore.

The *dhow* was the traditional boat used by pearl divers. Dhow-building is still an important industry today. In fact dhows still ply the waters between Bahrain and Saudi Arabia, providing basic taxi transport for very reasonable rates. Dhows are built from imported teak or mangrove wood along with local acacia, and a visit to a building site is a rewarding experience.

Famous entertainers often chose Bahrain as part of their itinerary when on performing tours. We attended musical concerts, ballets and plays, making a weekend of each event, eating at our favorite restaurants and staying in first-class hotels.

On the outskirts of the city, pleasant corners such as the country club provided havens in leafy-green garden surroundings where friends could meet for a delicious meal or a quiet rendezvous. This small island offered some of the pleasures which were not available in the Kingdom, and so a weekend in Bahrain was a welcome respite from the tedium of work.

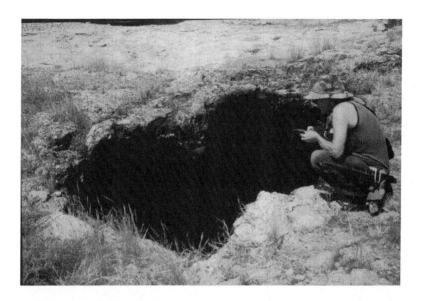

Mouth of Mossy Dahl.

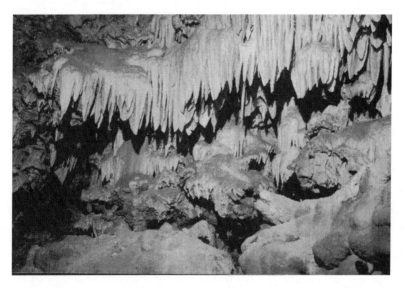

Inside the Mossy Dahl.

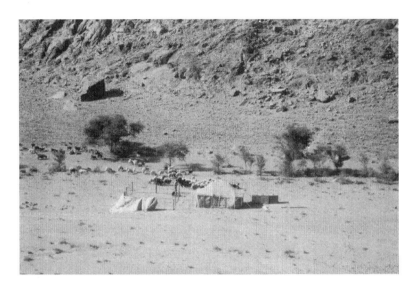

Bedouin tent and sheep, near Hail 1996.

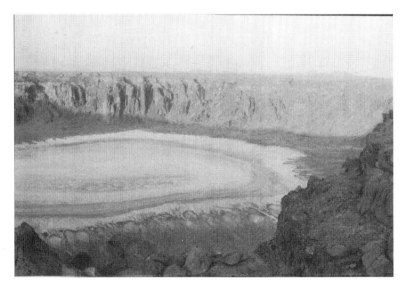

The Wabah Crater, west of Riyadh, 1992.

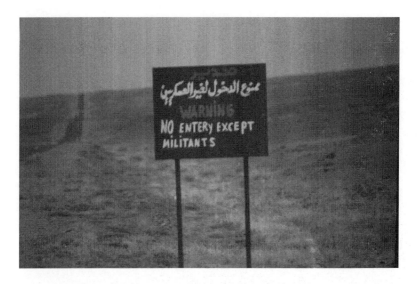

Sign in the desert east of Tabuk, 1995.

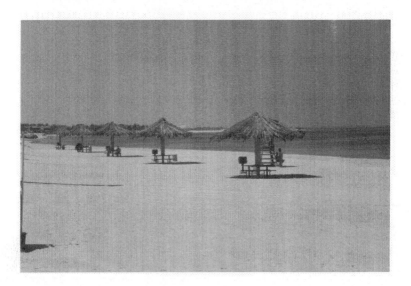

Beachfront Ras Tanura, 1992.

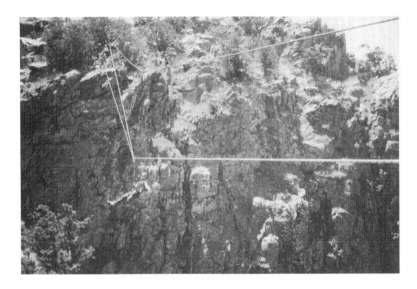

Rappelling in the Asir range, 1998.

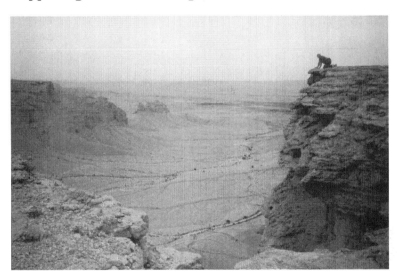

Rappelling with Boy Scouts on the Riyadh escarpment.

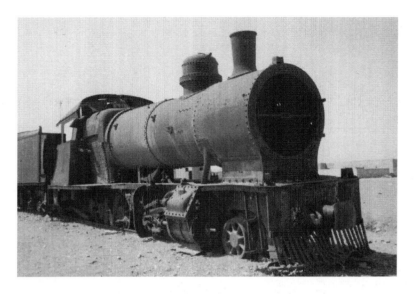

Train from the era of Lawrence of Arabia, Hijaz.

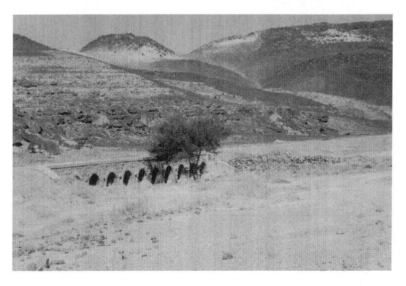

Culvert along the Hijaz railway, 1994.

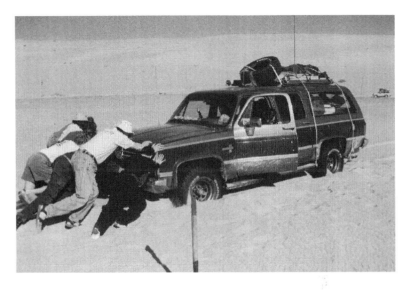

Stuck in the Rub Al Khali, 1994.

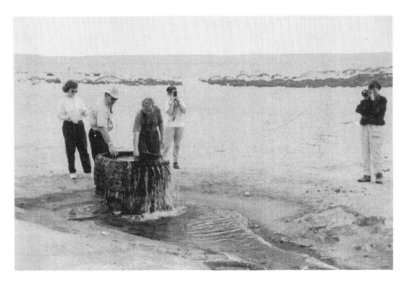

Sulphurous spring, Rub Al Khali 1998.

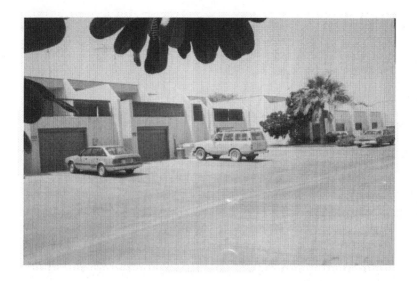

Driftwood Court, where I lived for five years.

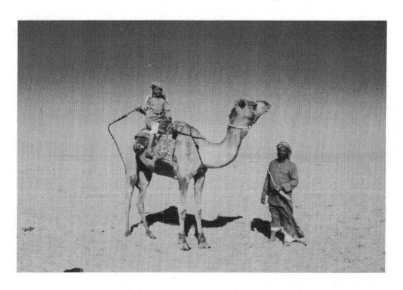

Kind Bedouin near Najran, south of Hofuf, 1994.

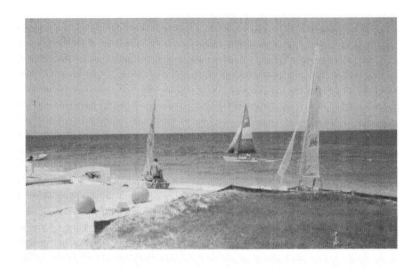

Enjoying a day at the Yacht Club, Ras Tanura, 1995.

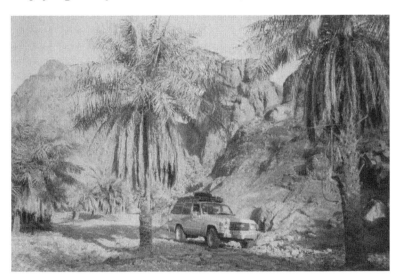

Camping near Buraydah, 1996.

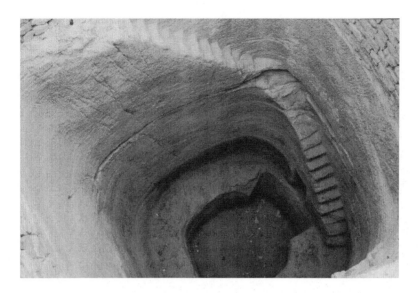

Nabatean well near Sakaka, Al Jawf, 1997.

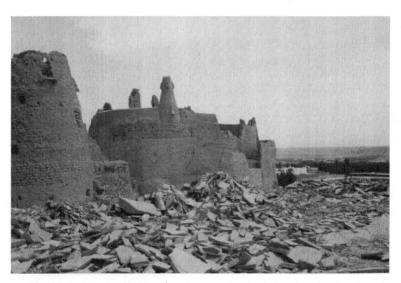

Famous ruins, Sakaka, 1997.

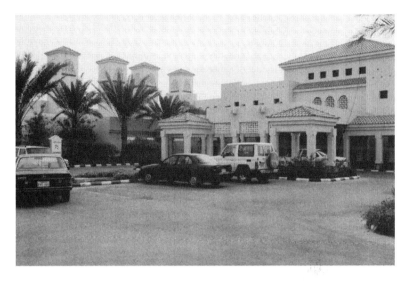

Five star hotel, Sakaka, Al Jawf, 1997.

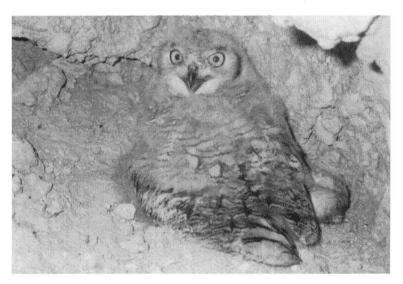

Owlet under rock overhang on jebel, Ma'aqala, 1997.

14 - GOLD, FRANKINCENSE AND MY FIRST CHRISTMAS

MY FIRST WHITE CHRISTMAS had been in Switzerland. Snowflakes breathed a white eiderdown over everything while church bells rang and rustic streetlights glowed. It was a Hallmark event.

The desert was every bit as blindingly white as snow, but December in Arabia was to be very different from the Christmas season anywhere else in the world. In a country where you never thought to add 'if it's fine,' when planning any outdoor activity, it even rained. The dust-clogged drains overflowed. Water backed up until the streets of Rahima were flooded. Now I understood why the curbs were so high and why you had to climb steps to enter the stores.

A few weeks before December 25th, our close-knit community exploded into action. 'Holiday,' was code for 'Christmas'. There were holiday parties, holiday trees, holiday cakes, holiday lights and holiday *suqs*.

The latter were bazaar-like stalls at a special weekend market set up in the Surf House, with all the excitement of Christmas shopping back home. There you could buy handmade candles and paper, specialized cards, patchwork quilts, Christmas ornaments of all kinds, stained-glass kaleidoscopes, angels, fridge magnets and many other beautifully crafted items, things which had been made by dependent wives throughout the year for this very event. Gold teaspoons, packaged with small chunks of frankincense and myrrh, were a touching reminder of the reason for the season.

Even Saudi Arabs got involved, the women buying up treasures such as tree decorations, colored lights and tinsel. They loved the sparkle of the celebrations as much as anybody and shrugged off the stern restrictions placed on the event by the company administration.

Christmas Day had once been a company holiday, but over the years since the Saudi Arabs took full management of the company, more and more restrictions had been placed on it until the day was declared a regular work day like any other.

One year a memo went to all employees, forbidding Christmas trees to be placed in house windows. Another year, 'you can have lights but they must be *down low.*' The next year lights were forbidden altogether.

Many people smuggled Christmas trees into Kingdom in their shipments. Some went to great lengths to disguise them, placing pieces in various boxes to reduce the chance of recognition by customs officials. Gerry was held up in Customs once, over a Christmas tree.

"I must take it," said the official. "It's a Christmas tree. It's *haraam,* forbidden."

"It's not a Christmas tree, it's an artificial house plant," Gerry argued.

"It's a Christmas tree."

"It's not."

They sat there drinking tea and arguing for half an hour before the official gave in.

"OK take it," he said.

The crazy thing was that you could buy Christmas trees in Al Khobar. You could dial a certain phone number and whisper the word, 'Christmas tree'. You would then be told where to drive to and would be met by a van. When the coast was clear you would hand over your money and take delivery of your very own Christmas tree.

Later on, artificial Christmas trees could be purchased in stores in Rahima. Almost anything one desired could be obtained in Kingdom for a price.

Weeks before Christmas the parties began. Certain houses were renowned for their annual gatherings, with hundreds of expatriates from Ras Tanura and other camps passing through in an evening. For some employees it was the only time they got to socialize with each other. A highlight was the appearance of a Filipino choir, which sang with gusto and collected money for charity.

Everyone gave cards by the dozen—even to folks they saw every day at work. That seemed strange to me, an Australian used to sending cards by mail only to those friends seldom visited, but I soon entered the spirit of things and strung cards up in my apartment as merrily as my neighbors. It was depressing to have to pack them all away along with the Christmas decorations after the 'holiday season'.

Christmas Day in my first year fell on a weekend so it was automatically a holiday. Aramco was very quiet. Many people had gone on short leave back to their home countries. I was invited to lunch with friends in Dhahran, where a whole turkey was deep fried in a steel bucket over a gas burner from the school science lab.

The turkey was huge. It was suspended in the boiling oil on great steel skewers, also from the science lab. It was the best turkey I'd ever tasted.

I also went with friends to a Christmas concert in an auditorium in Dhahran, where we were held spellbound by music, short plays and the enactment of the first Christmas in Bethlehem. The musical talent in Aramco was unsurpassed and there was even a bell choir, the likes of which I had never heard before.

One year, just before Christmas, word spread that there was real Christmas fabric available in a certain store in Khobar. I went to see for myself. Sure enough, in the back of the store were two large rolls of fabric, one green and one red, with all the symbols of Christmas around the borders—plum puddings, little churches, trees, Santas, sleighs and reindeer.

"How on earth did you get this into Kingdom?" I asked the shop owner.

"When I ordered the last shipment," he said with a grin, "I told them, 'Put it inside. Put it *way* inside!'"

The fabric made beautiful tablecloths. It was sold out within days.

Just before Christmas each year a special visitor would arrive and make his way to the school building. Dressed in a bright red suit and wearing his own long luxurious white beard, Santa delighted the children and passed out small gifts. His job at Christmas time was seasonal; the rest of the year he worked for the Personnel Department, beard and all.

In the early days of Aramco, Christmas celebrations were the norm and even the Saudi Arabs entered into the spirit of things. There was no attempt to hide any part of Christmas, either the Story itself or the secular celebrations. Real camels and barn animals were used in a pageant held in a playing field in Dhahran.

As time went on and restrictions grew, they seemed to produce the opposite effect from that which the instigators intended. Instead of being watered down and broken up, Christmas became even more a symbol of rightness and importance and welded an already tightly-knit community even closer together. Here, far away from loved ones and the freedoms we enjoyed in our home communities, we relied upon each other for support and courage.

15 - FIRST REPAT

ACCORDING TO company regulations, I waited a whole year for my first 'repat', or annual leave. As I was also entitled to attach some leave from my second year's allowance it would be the longest vacation I could ever have with Aramco.

I arranged my "exit re-entry" visa with excitement. My parents decided to join me in a trip around Europe. It was their first time in the Northern Hemisphere and we enjoyed a rail tour around much of Europe before I had to return to work.

My parents were able to get a stop-over in Bahrain on their way back to Australia. They were still on a high and very excited about visiting Bahrain, even in the hundred-plus degree heat of early July. Rob and I met them at the airport and took them to a hotel we had booked earlier.

Several friends had said they would take the opportunity to cross the causeway and meet them, including Suheim, and Mohamed Suwani, Kathy's Saudi Arabian colleague from work. The Suwani family was rich and powerful; they were the ones who owned the large ship in a center island on the road leading into Ras Tanura. Mohamed, or Suwani as we called him, frequently used his family's influence to advantage.

It was Thursday night and we were in a restaurant waiting for our meals when a disheveled Suheim burst in. He had come over the causeway the previous night, he said, and had stayed in a hotel, but when he woke up in the morning his car was gone. He'd spent all day looking for it, to no avail.

"I even asked the police," he lamented, "but they aren't interested in helping me."

I felt sorry for the young man, and even more so when I learned that his plant ID had been in the glove box. As well as my assistant in the Rehab unit, he was a volunteer fire fighter and as such had been given a special permit to enter the refinery.

A plant ID should never be taken out of the country, and Suheim would be in deep trouble if he did not find it before returning to work. Suwani listened silently to Suheim's tale of woe.

"Leave it with me," he said suddenly and strode out of the room. A few minutes later he returned.

The evening proceeded with lively conversation and even Suheim began to relax, when a waiter came into the room.

"There's a phone call for you, sir," he said to Suwani.

Suheim's car had been found by the police at another hotel, and Suheim was awash with relief when he realized that both his car and plant ID were safe and well.

"The Chief of Police is a friend of mine," Suwani explained. "I asked him to find the car for you."

Next day we drove around the *suqs*, and explored Arad Fort. It was an impressive sight but the warm day sapped our energy.

In the late afternoon another friend of Kathy's, Arouf, joined us, accompanied by his grandfather. The old man took an instant liking to my father as both men sported white beards, and he rambled on in broken English for an hour or so, delighting my parents. He had obviously been drinking something which loosened his tongue considerably, and bade my father to come visit him anytime in Saudi Arabia.

"You are my brother," he crooned. "My house is your house. Anytime you want to come, just stay as long as you want."

Suwani had organized a traditional *kabsa* meal for my parents in a friend's home, another middle-eastern experience. Too soon it was time to leave. We rushed them from the taxi to the check-in line at the airport but after they had completed formalities at the desk, to their chagrin, security guards prevented them from returning to say their good-byes. At this point, Suwani arrived in his car.

"Where are your parents?" he asked, and I quickly explained.

"One moment," he said, and boldly walked into the restricted area.

After a private word with the security guards, he walked my parents back with him through the gate. To this day my parents are convinced that there is nothing Suwani can't do.

With my parents gone I began to feel depressed. Strange, I thought, I've never been prone to depression. Friends laughed.

"It's a very common reaction after a first repat," I was told. "Wait a couple of weeks and you'll get over it."

At about this time Kathy left Arabia. She had been very homesick and had also been battling an illness which was hard to manage. Much as she loved 'all things Arabic', she felt she could not stay so I sadly bid her goodbye.

Still in temporary housing, I wondered if a new house might lift my spirits and provide an incentive to stay longer with the company. My finances were beginning to look healthier and another year or two with Aramco would really help the mortgage on my house in Australia.

Points accrued due to time worked plus my grade code put me only halfway up the female housing list so I didn't hold out too much hope of securing the house of the month—a roomy two-storey bachelor apartment in Driftwood Court, the classiest complex for singles, on the beachfront. I put my name down anyway.

During Eid I opted to stay on camp, allowing my finances to recover from the trip to Europe. And I won the house! Most of the females ahead of me on the housing list had gone away for the week and had been either too busy to bid or absent when the housing offer had been posted.

I had mixed feelings about winning the bid. It would be harder to save if I spent more on rent. On the other hand it would be more comfortable in a larger house and I'd be more inclined to stay longer.

So I accepted the house. A tingle of anticipation ran through me as I walked in for the first time as the new occupant. The apartment was open-plan and very spacious. A combined dining/lounge area, guest bathroom and kitchen filled the ground floor, and there was plenty of storage under the stairs. The lounge room opened into a small grassed courtyard.

On the upper floor, a large bedroom overlooked the lounge with its cathedral ceiling. Off the bedroom opened a private bathroom, and another door led onto a large balcony, which looked across the car park to the Arabian Gulf beyond. Under the large balcony was a lock-up garage.

There had to be a housewarming! I busied myself with plans for feeding and entertaining guests and arranged for several to be billeted out with other friends in RT.

The party was fun. My new apartment buzzed with the sounds of happiness and when everyone had gone I stopped to reflect. People here seemed closer to each other than in most other communities I'd lived in. Perhaps because we were all displaced persons we pulled together to help and to nurture each other as much as we could. I'd found a new family. The blues were gone and I was back to normal.

I was now in the upper level of singles' accommodation. Those who were high-grade employees, such as doctors and dentists, lived here, as did those who had earned their status by working for the company for many years.

Some nick-named it Sin City. A few residents lived unashamedly with partners. Others, married to spouses in their home countries, chose partners of convenience while they were in Kingdom. There were also those who were allegedly gay.

And there was even, so the rumors went, Ras Tanura's very own prostitute. Everyone seemed to know—Brianna frequently had men staying overnight, and she was often seen disappearing over the causeway to Bahrain with a man, sometimes even a Saudi Arab, in tow. She was a pretty brunette, always dressed to kill, and had no shortage of cash.

The Darts Club, the front for a night club of sorts, offered door prizes at their club meetings. The winner one day won a night out with Brianna—and the winner was an upstanding young new hire.

All the housewives who heard of it were horrified.

"Don't go," they implored him. "*Just don't go!*" I never heard if he followed their advice or not.

There was one single female on camp who terrified me. I would go out of my way to avoid her. Tessa was Irish and had connections with the IRA. Every man in her holiday pictures from Ireland was shielding his face from the camera. It was also said that whenever she went through Heathrow airport she was called aside for questioning.

Tessa was a mannish-looking female, whose current boyfriend was a married man with a wife at home in Britain. Although he wanted to break off with Tessa he was afraid to do so. The last boyfriend to dump her had incurred a most impressive display of wrath. She had smashed several cars in the car park, amongst other misdemeanors, on her rampage. The lady was a monster when drunk, and drunk she often was.

Tessa didn't own a boat but belonged to the yacht club anyway, as did several other non-boat-owners in Ras Tanura. Membership entitled one to entry to the premises at any time, and use of the private beach in front of the club. Yacht Club members also attended regular functions, including the annual Yacht Club ball.

The afternoon I attended my first annual general meeting of the yacht club, I saw Tessa in action. She was indignant because she had not received a personal invitation to the ball and had therefore not been able to apply to attend in time.

The Commodore courteously explained that it had been decided not to send out personal invitations that year, but to advertise only in the yacht club newsletter. It was not good enough for Tessa. She argued, shouted, interrupted and turned the meeting into a shambles. The Commodore didn't stand a chance. I was trembling by the end of her tirade.

Tessa's boyfriend later went to the Commodore and apologized for her behavior. He explained that Tessa had certainly been aware of the impending Yacht club ball and had wanted to go to both the Yacht Club and the Golf Club functions in Bahrain. He had promised to take her to one of these functions in Bahrain but not both, and had asked her to choose which one. She had chosen the Golf Club ball. Why she decided to make an issue of the Yacht Club invitations will forever be a mystery.

One year, at a Golf Club ball in Bahrain, Tessa had had more than her share of potent libations when she caught sight of the Yacht Club Commodore for that year, who was also attending the ball. Philip was an Englishman, the most polite, pleasant individual one could hope to meet. Tessa stomped over to him and stamped on his foot.

"Why don't you get back to the Yacht Club where you belong," she hissed.

The only reason that Tessa's employment was not terminated was that she had connections in high places. Even the Arabs were afraid of her! Nevertheless, we heard that she had finally been given a transfer to another department as her boss had had enough of her tantrums.

At times one could be forgiven for wondering if everyone in Aramco was a misfit. Certainly, people in Aramco were different. To accept the conditions of residence, vastly different from the countries most of us hailed from, demanded a certain degree of compliance. And the people we were when we arrived were different to the people we became, as we lived in the melting pots of the camps.

After I moved into my new home, life began to change in other ways. Another therapist was allocated to our physical therapy unit. Deanna was a young Irish lass, tall and strikingly beautiful, and she took our hearts by storm. Her wide blue eyes and full mouth smiled constantly. She was also a skilful therapist who soon found her place in the clinic.

But it was too good to last. As the months went by it became clear that Deanna was unhappy. There were few people of her age in RT and most weekends she went to Dhahran where there were more activities for young people. When she asked for a transfer I understood and supported her proposal, and soon Deanna took up duties in the Dhahran clinic.

One evening I found myself sitting next to another Australian physiotherapist at a function in the British Aerospace compound. Pat was interested in working for Aramco and I encouraged her to apply for the soon-to-be-vacant position at RT. She did so, although it was several months before she arrived and started work with me.

Pat and I shared the same work ethic as well as many common dreams and aspirations; we started in-service education classes involving just the two of us, and explored new techniques and methods of treatment. Seldom did we have a disagreement and when we did it was quickly resolved.

With two therapists the waiting lists diminished and fewer complaints rolled in. Those were good days, when we pinned cartoons on the office wall and chuckled at each other's jokes. Occasionally we came into the office during difficult treatments to indulge in 'silent screams.'

Pat had one big problem—she was a heavy smoker. We were both concerned about the effect on her health and she determined to give it up. I admired her strength and consistency even on the worst days. She would often come into the office with a strained look on her face, saying, "I would give anything for a cigarette right now!" With the help of nicotine patches and lots of determination, the cravings gradually became less and less.

She also had support from a certain electrician from the British Aerospace compound, who visited every weekend and disliked the smoking habit. Pat had known Barry in her previous job but they had been just friends. Now they began seeing each other seriously, although they had frequent disagreements.

"I sorted out the CD's again," Pat would say. "As if he's leaving!" Laughter hid her pain. And then they'd be back together again.

The credit card debt I had incurred with the building of my cottage in Australia was gone now and the rent was fully covering the mortgage repayments. I could ease up a little on my tight budget and began to furnish my apartment in RT.

Middle Eastern antiques had held little attraction for me early on but now I had begun to appreciate them. Gradually my apartment was transformed. A large copper pot filled with brightly colored silk poppies stood on one corner of the lounge room, line drawings of camels and Bedouin tents hung on my walls along with hand-woven rugs, and a potted tree stood in another corner opposite the piano. My apartment became a peaceful haven.

Each nationality hired by Aramco had a different package of conditions. Due to our small numbers, Australians were on the British Sterling payroll. We received a lower rate of pay than either the Canadians or Americans, but we got an extra month's pay per year. The vacation allowances and the shipping allowances were less also.

I grew to deeply appreciate my friends of all nationalities, and stayed in contact with many of them after leaving Arabia. The American women on camp were notable for their 'big hair', perfect makeup and coordinated garments. They shopped at Sears and J.C. Penney department stores when in the USA and through Land's End and L.L. Bean catalogues when they were not.

Many of them jangled armfuls of gold bangles, and layers of neck chains—the precious twenty-two carat metal could be had for virtually the world price of gold. These beautiful women were unfailingly polite and very, very kind.

16 - IN TROUBLE

IT HAPPENED ONE sunny Thursday, in Al Khobar outside the Safeway supermarket during prayer time. Katrina, another Physical Therapist from Australia, had arrived a few weeks previously and we sat face to face on a large concrete block at the edge of the car park, chatting about life in Arabia. Katrina looked over my shoulder with sudden alarm.

"There's a Suburban circling around the car park and it's full of *mutawas*, religious police!" she gasped.

"Never mind," I reassured her. "Just ignore them. We aren't doing anything wrong."

A moment later Katrina's eyes widened again.

"Oh no! They've stopped and they're coming over—and there's a policeman with them!"

That indeed was bad news, for a policeman meant serious business. By now I could hear shouting. I thought quickly. If the *mutawa* were reasonable and willing to talk, I would show them an official newsletter from the company in Arabic and English which explained the dress code and other company policies, to prove that we were complying with regulations. We could also stand our ground and demand an official be sent from Aramco Government Affairs to assist us. *Mutawas* were not allowed to touch a woman and in that regard we were better off than if we had been men.

Now there were also plenty of witnesses—people were coming from everywhere to see what the commotion was about. The shouting had increased and it was obvious that the *mutawas* were anything but reasonable.

"Go home! Where is your *abaya*? Go home! You are ugly!" The figure leading the group towards us bellowed over and over.

"Look at me!" I hissed to Katrina. "Just keep on talking. Ignore him! Don't even look at him."

We tried to continue our conversation as he approached, each keeping our gaze fixed firmly on the other as the volume of the harangue escalated. The *mutawa* must have been shouting for at least five minutes while the crowd gathered. The man was in no mind to listen to me or to look at the paper about Aramco code of dress even if I had tried to show it to him.

I was beginning to wonder how much longer this could go on when all of a sudden, like a tap turned off, he stopped and marched back to the vehicle with the others trailing behind. The lone policeman trailed uncomfortably at the rear of the procession.

"We won!" I said, my knees trembling.

Later that afternoon back in camp, I parked the car near Rob's house and opened the trunk to get something out. Suddenly a voice behind me echoed,

"Go home! Go home!"

I spun around. It was a neighbor, grinning from ear to ear. His wife had been in town that morning and had witnessed our ordeal.

It was not the only experience I had with *mutawas*. While walking down the main street of Khobar one afternoon with Dean and Maria, a prayer call started and a vehicle drew level with us, a loudspeaker blaring. The man holding the loudspeaker at the car window was glaring right at us.

"Don't look at him, just keep on walking!" whispered Maria frantically. Dean had already disappeared. Soon the *mutawa* also moved on.

As Dean and Maria had told me, if a woman ever attracted the attention of a *mutawa* it was best for the man to have nothing to do with her. The most a *mutawa* could do to a woman was to yell at her but a man could be manhandled and dragged off to jail. I never heard of whips being used on women in the Eastern Province.

One Christmas Day in Kingdom Rob invited me over to his place, along with his son and daughter-in-law who were visiting from Canada. We had all decided to go across to Rahima for a walk and I had not had a chance to change from my dress into pants and top. It was a long dress with long sleeves but it was form-fitting and, horrors, had a waist.

Two young *mutawa* approached quickly and I moved away from Rob's side but it was too late. They had seen that we were together and spoke with him. It is usually the fault of the man if a woman misbehaves, for he is her controller and should see to it that she toes the line. One of the *mutawa* pointed at me.

"She should wear something!" he said.

Rob raised his eyebrows.

"Really?"

"How long have you lived here? Maybe you don't know the rules."

"I've lived here for thirteen years. I know the rules. Long sleeves and long skirt. No problem."

The young men's English was not good and Rob did not volunteer that he spoke reasonable Arabic. The mutawas struggled for a few minutes to convey their meaning before giving up and walking off. This experience amused rather than frightened me.

On another occasion I was sitting at the photography shop in Rahima, waiting for a passport photo, when a *mutawa* entered. He was big and burly with a thick shaggy beard, and gave me an ugly glance before shoving aside an Indian customer at the desk and speaking gruffly to the shop attendant.

I had just bought a mop and seriously considered allowing the handle to slip down behind his ankle, so he'd trip on it as he turned around to leave. I almost regretted not having done so when I later asked the shop attendant what the *mutawa* had said.

"He told me I should not let ladies sit in the shop," was his reply.

Mutawas were not my only source of trouble. One day I noticed a painful, red swelling on the inside of my left knee. It grew larger and more painful until I had trouble walking.

I showed it to Rob.

"Hell!" he said. "You'd better see a doctor."

I chose Doctor Peter Burg because he was a friend. He was also the only American doctor on staff. He was very pleasant socially, enjoyed a party and a good laugh, and as a doctor he was meticulous although his bedside manner could be gruff.

"I'll put you on antibiotics," he said, "But if this doesn't clear up in a week's time come back and we'll lance it."

I gasped.

"What? *Mafi amalia*, no surgery?" he joked.

A few days later I discovered that even coasting along on my bicycle was impossible. Bending the knee was excruciating. I had to use a walking stick from my stock cupboard at work to get around. During the morning Peter called.

"I saw you limping to work this morning. You had better come over to my office as soon as you can."

When Peter's nurse saw my leg she grimaced.

That's the biggest abscess I've ever seen."

"Thanks," I said wryly.

Peter drew up some local anesthetic in a syringe and plunged it, so it seemed, right into the middle of the abscess.

"OWWWWW!" I yelled.

"Quiet!" he ordered.

"But it hurts! It hurts!"

"It does not! Lie down," he growled and stabbed the abscess with a lancet.

I was sweating by now, driving my thumbs through the palm of the nurse's hand.

"It does so hurt!" I yelled again.

And then it was over. I panted while the throbbing wound was drained and bandaged, and gingerly stood up with my walking stick again.

Peter smiled. "There! That wasn't so bad, was it?"

I rolled my eyes.

"I think you'd better take the rest of the day off," he continued. "You should rest that leg today. You should come in and have it dressed every day for a while too, until it stops draining and the edges heal over."

I hobbled back to the department, but by the time I'd finished treating the waiting patients I was unable to cancel and did the bookwork, it was closing time anyway.

I was seldom ill and it was just as well—there was nobody to cover for me if I had been sick. Large numbers of referrals were flooding in and I did my best to see them all as soon as possible. The schedule was a continual balancing act, between new patients hoping for immediate appointments and 'no shows'.

The latter were patients who failed to keep their appointments, either because they decided they didn't need any more treatment and didn't bother to cancel, or simply waltzed in later and expected to be seen then.

"Sorry," I'd say, "You're late. I'll have to reschedule you."

"But I am here!" they would cry. "I have an appointment!"

"No, you *had* an appointment, which you didn't keep," I learned to say firmly. "I was ready for you and you didn't come. Now I have other patients and I am busy. We'll have to make you another appointment."

It was hard to be tough on people from a culture where time was unimportant. Their world view was people and event based, rather than time based. For that reason there was no shame in coming late to an appointment, a meeting, or a social gathering. The important thing was that they came, not that they were late.

But was I was the one who had it all wrong? When I looked at Western logic and saw how screwed up we get over punctuality and how stressed out we become over schedules and work volume, I wondered if it was worth the fuss. Rob used to say that Western logic, Oriental logic and Arabic logic were all at right angles to each other. Still, we had to function as a unit in an organization based on Western logic and there were rules to keep.

The Saudi Arabian women were sometimes impatient but generally they were a lot more flexible than their male counterparts. After all, they were used to waiting. They spent their lives waiting—waiting for fathers and brothers to take them somewhere, waiting in shops, waiting for transport to hospitals and schools. They are forbidden to drive themselves.

I came to deeply appreciate my female Arabian friends. Some could be excruciatingly shy, speaking to me through their veils even when alone with me, a Western woman. I felt honored when a woman would discard her veil and speak face to face with me in confidence.

They shared with me their thoughts, their customs and their humor, and I learned a lot about how they lived. Some wore odd things under their *abayas*, such as their husband's pajamas, and in summer they would all come in dripping of perspiration from head to toe. Why *does* a society dress its women in black in temperatures which typically soar over a hundred degrees day after day, while men waft around in coolest white?

Women varied in appearance, from those with heavy, dark features to fair-complexioned. Some were ravishing beauties, others very plain. I enjoyed meeting all of them. Sometimes, when in a market place or out on the street, I'd be rushed by a shapeless black figure, babbling in rapid Arabic, who turned out to be a patient or ex-patient. If only everyone could have the opportunity to meet and dialogue with those of differing cultures there would be fewer misunderstandings.

17 - THE BIGGEST OASIS

AN HOUR AND a half on the road south of Dhahran sprawls Al Hofuf in the area of Al Hasa, one of the largest oases of Arabia. The lush greenery is a feast to the eyes after the stark glare of sun on sand. It is said that habitation has been continuous here for around three thousand, two hundred years, making this the oldest continuously inhabited city on earth.

The Turks used Hofuf as their headquarters from 1871 to 1913, when it was seized by Abdul Aziz Ibn Saud, and it became part of the nation of Saudi Arabia in 1932.

There are around three million date palms in the Al Hasa Oasis, watered by an intricate system of irrigations channels and fed from a vast underground aquifer; this water is very old and is said to have drained from the western part of the Arabian peninsula. Geologically the Arabian Peninsula is tilted, with the lower end being at the Arabian Gulf in the east.

In the town itself many of the ancient buildings have stood the test of time. These structures consist mainly of mud, with hardwood reinforcements most likely imported from nearby Africa. The roofs were made of palm fronds, palm trees and mud. In places horse hair was also used as a binding agent.

The old fort, *Qasr Ibrahim,* or *Qasr Kut* as it is also called, dates from the mid 1550's, its walls thirty feet high and six feet thick in parts. It was built by the Ottoman Governor Al-Burayki in the mid 1550's and renovated by the Saudi Arabian Governor Ibrahim Ibn 'Ufaysan in the early 1800's. The Mosque of Ibrahim, or Al-Qubbah Mosque, was built within the walls and also dates from the early 1800's. It is a wonderful example of Moslem architecture.

Qasr Ibrahim is not often open to the public, but the Arabian Natural History group in Ras Tanura had been able to arrange a tour. Our group, numbering about forty, spent two and a half hours in an Aramco bus on desert highways before we pulled up in front of the fort. We straggled out of the bus, walked through the huge gates in the wall and were met by a pleasant young government officer in a clean white *thowb.*

"You are welcome to walk around wherever you wish," he said. "Please feel free to ask any questions."

I approached him hesitantly.

"I understand that we are not allowed to photograph anything," I said.

"That's right," he said. "Today there will be no photography."

"Is there ever a chance to take photographs?" I asked. "I mean, on other days?"

He stood quietly for a moment, obviously struggling between duty and his sense of hospitality. At last he smiled.

"Well, if you are very quick!" he said.

I needed no further invitation and dashed back to the bus to grab my camera. Quickly I hurried around the compound, trying to look inconspicuous while taking as many photographs as I could.

One of the main reasons for coming to Hofuf was its markets—genuine local markets with only the infrequent expatriate worker. In the vast area under cover one could buy anything Arabic, and I loved poking around in its musty corners.

As well as everyday clothing and food supplies, antique stalls stocked Bedouin jewelry, daggers, swords, coffee pots, old firearms, incense burners, rugs, camel stools and other furniture. The smell of spices and old leather was intoxicating. Sweating Indians forged metal, men stitched moccasins, women sold baskets.

In the animal markets we found birds in cages, sheep, goats, chickens and camels—all were for sale for the right price. I could watch the camels for hours. Men haggled over prices and when a sale was made, the animal was disabled by tying its legs in a folded position so it could not stand.

Then ropes were attached to a sling under the bawling beast's belly. A crane lifted it skyward and deposited it gently into a waiting pick-up. Working camels, racing camels and camels destined for cooking pots were all there. Baby camels waited on spindly legs with their mothers, calling intermittently through the din and the dust.

Young men stood by offering camel rides for eager expatriates for a small fee. One coaxed a grumbling animal to its knees and I climbed awkwardly onto a seat behind its hump. As it stood, I feared I would slide off its back and then suddenly there I was—on top of the world! We ambled awkwardly around the enclosure until the young Saudi Arab whistled gently and my mount and I descended shakily toward solid ground.

After exploring the fort and the markets we clambered onto the bus again, ready for another adventure. On the edge of the *Hasa* oasis, at *Jebel Qara*, the *Ghar Al-Hashshab* (arrow maker) caves yawn from part of the escarpment that runs north-south.

Erosion has formed deep clefts in the rock, making passageways that lead to the caves. It is cool here, a favorite place for picnics, and in one of these caves is a pottery. Earthen vessels of all shapes and sizes are formed on wheels there, then baked in a low-fire kiln and sold.

"Be very careful if you buy one," I had been warned. "They are great decorative pieces but never bring water anywhere near them—they will dissolve."

Near these caves was one of my favorite camping places. There, where red cliffs meet, is a niche where three or four vehicles can park unseen. Several of us camped here one Christmas Eve and each family brought part of the meal, making a full Christmas dinner with all the trimmings.

As we started to eat, three Saudi Arabs arrived in a pick-up, planning to have a picnic of their own. We did the sociable thing and invited them to join us. Now there was *kabsa* on our menu, and turkey and plum sauce on theirs!

18 - BLACK PEARLS

"I'M GOING ON a fantastic camping trip over the Eid break!" Tanya was excited. "My friend Luke is taking a group of us to the meteorite crater in the Rub Al Khali. And guess what? There's room for you too, if you want to come!"

My heart raced. What an opportunity! I had heard of this site, deep in the desert of southern Arabia, where a meteorite had landed in 1863. It had come blazing across the sky one night during a thunderstorm, convincing the local Bedouin that the end of the world was nigh. In the morning they discovered a huge crater in the sand. The whole area was strewn with what they assumed to be black pearls—shiny beads of fused sand which had formed in the intense heat.

The meteorite had broken into two pieces, a rabbit-sized piece which the explorer Philby took to the Museum in London, and a large piece weighing two and a half tons which is now located at the Riyadh Natural History Museum. There was still apparently a crater at the site, amazing since the desert winds had been working away at it for well over a hundred years.

"I'd love to come!" I answered eagerly.

The next few weeks went quickly, and before long we were away. Three vehicles embarked on the trip—a Suburban and two Land Cruisers, with thirteen passengers in all.

I rode with Luke, Tanya and Amy in the Suburban, a heavy rig with a lifter kit adding fifteen centimetres above the original suspension. We packed it with camping equipment, food, water, and jerry cans of fuel.

Each vehicle was equipped with a global positioning system, which we kept hidden away until we reached the limit of mapped roads and the last of the checkpoints. At this time GPS units, mobile phones, walkie-talkie radios and even the taking of photographs were banned in the Kingdom for security reasons.

I had once mentioned the Rub Al Khali, the 'Empty Quarter' which filled much of the southern half of Saudi Arabia, to an English patient.

"Where's that?" he asked.

I was astounded.

"Don't you know?"

"No," he replied. "I have no interest in seeing anything in this god-forsaken country. I go to work and I come home again. I don't even bother going to *Khobar*, I can get everything I need in *Rahima*."

Unbelievable, I thought. How could a person find themselves in this amazing country and close their eyes to its treasures?

We did not enter the *Rub Al Khali* lightly. Even in winter the desert can be deadly. Many have perished in this wild, white land, from their own foolishness or by mishap. Water, fuel and shelter are of prime importance, as well as a mechanically sound vehicle and good navigational skills. It pays to take more than one spare tire and have at least one companion vehicle.

We reached the Aramco *Udailiyah* compound on the first evening and stayed the night with friends. The next morning we sallied south, jolting along desert tracks under the blazing sun. A stony plain stretched ahead of us to a horizon of small hills against the sky, and after the village of *Yabriin* the tracks ended and the dunes began.

There had been some early rain and a crust had formed on the sand. If our speed was up we skimmed over the sand but if we slowed down, a wheel would break through the crust and we'd be bogged. The drivers took turns leading, although the following vehicles had to make their own tracks so their wheels did not sink down in the soft tracks of those in front.

Time after time the vehicles sank in soft patches, wheels spinning. "Out with the sand mats! Everybody push!" With a rubber mat under each wheel and several people heaving on the rear bumper, we'd be underway again. Sometimes one rig could tow another out, using a long nylon rope. Sometimes all vehicles were stuck at once and everyone would work together, getting one van up on hard ground then using it to tow another out.

After some particularly good runs, we all got stuck again and someone went for the long rope.

"It's not here!" he shouted, "We must have left it at the last stop."

Everyone groaned. The men decided there was nothing for it but to take one vehicle and retrace the tracks to the area where we had last needed the rope. We girls talked, fidgeted, wrote in our diaries and read books. Over two hours passed before the men returned, with defeated looks on their faces.

"Couldn't find the rope anywhere," said Luke.

"Are we *sure* it isn't in the truck?" asked one of the girls.

She went to the back of the truck, flung open both doors—and there was the rope! We made jokes about men who could not find anything unless it was right under their noses, and made camp beside the nearest dune.

Halfway through the next morning we arrived at *Nadqan*—a couple of tin sheds, a goat pen, and a fuel truck selling gas at double the price of that in town. Small children stared at us open-mouthed as we got out and stretched our legs. They pointed across to a decent looking gravel road.

"That road comes from *Harad* in the north," they said. "Why didn't you come that way?"

Groans filled the air again.

"You mean we went through all that sand for nothing?"

Luke grinned.

"Well, it was a very interesting experience, don't you think? Wouldn't it have been boring if we'd come straight here by the road?"

He stepped backward to avoid Ron, who suddenly attacked him.

From *Nadqan* we raced at a great rate across gravel plains and low sand dunes. After a late lunch, as we relaxed in the shade of the vehicles, a battered old pickup pulled alongside and two Bedouin men got out. I held my breath. The Al Murra tribe were known for their hostility and some expatriates claimed to have been shot at while passing through the Murra territory.

However, Luke, who grew up in Aramco, was fluent in Arabic and soon discovered that our visitors needed help. They had been trying for four days to get the wheel off a large truck so they could change the tire, but their tools were pitifully inadequate.

"Let's go, guys!" Luke said.

The men gathered all the tools they could find from the backs of the vehicles and were soon back, jubilant.

"We got it off with two jacks and some WD 40," said Luke. "Now they can't do enough for us."

It was time to move on, but down the track our new friends were standing with a camel in colorful harness and we stopped to take photos. The Murra men motioned for us to take rides on the beast, so one by one we mounted the camel and took pictures of each other. It was a nice way to say "thank you."

The weather was clear and the nights very cold. I slept on an old army cot under a blanket of stars.

"I saw the Southern Cross last night," said Amy on the third morning.

"Impossible!" Tanya said.

"I *know* it was the Southern Cross," Amy insisted.

And she was correct. In February each year, we discovered, the Southern Cross is visible in the Northern Hemisphere, standing just above the horizon in an upright position.

We drove over countless dunes, carefully scouting around the edges before launching ourselves onto the slip faces, where we'd slowly coast in the loose sand to the bottom. When firm sand rose up below the wheels we'd accelerate and drive away.

Experienced drivers chose a speed that was not fast enough to make their vehicle airborne at the top of the slip-face, and not slow enough to become high-centered on it. Some of us were so nervous of the gradient on the slip face that we chose to get out of the vehicles and walk down the slopes.

On the eve of the third full day, two hundred miles from *Nadqan*, we reached the general area of the meteorite crater. Next morning we drove about in circles, trying to determine the exact locality from an old photograph. Suddenly, someone realized that all over the ground were black 'pearls.'

"It must be within half a mile!" I said. "The article I read said the pearls were scattered over a radius of about half a mile."

And then we saw it, or rather, them. There were two craters, one around twelve feet deep, the second one smaller, and we hurried out of the vehicles to gather samples.

"You can collect fragments of metal from the meteor with magnets," we'd been told. "Just put the magnet on one side of a plastic bag and drag it through the sand. When you find a piece of metal, turn the bag inside out, and then remove the magnet and the fragments will fall into the bag."

Satisfied with my collection of meteorite samples, I turned my attention to the black "pearls". Those which had been lying in the open, tumbling about in the wind, were quite weathered and dull but those just under the surface were black and shiny. They were very light-weight and I cracked one open to find a white, porous core.

For two hours we poked around in the craters, before regretfully piling into the four-wheel drives and heading homeward. It would be two solid days of driving before we reached Dhahran and another hour for me on the bus to Ras Tanura.

We plunged into the hot dry plains, speeding toward the dunes. This time we had to pick our way between the slip faces, finding gaps to climb on. The sun was high in the sky and there were no shadows to mark the edges of the slip faces when it happened—BANG!

We had hit a hard ridge at the leeward front of a dune and were airborne. Things flew across the cabin. Someone screamed. And then it was over. The Suburban was resting at a crazy angle and as we tumbled out of the vehicle the problem was clear. A broken axle!

"Ah no!" sighed Luke. "We're a couple of days from home and we can't fix this here. Let's take the fuel drums and bury them. We'll take what luggage we can but we'll have to leave some of it. Everyone will have to cram into the two other vehicles. I'm going to come back and try to repair it but I'm afraid if the Bedou find it they will strip it."

Once again we set off, but our high spirits had evaporated. Tanya and I squeezed into Ron's Land Cruiser, experiencing a much rougher ride than we'd had in the Suburban.

Ron seemed to ignore the boundaries of the track, sometimes driving on the track and sometimes off, and it was no surprise when a tire blew out. A few miles down the track another tire blew. Finally Ron admitted that he had long distance glasses which he had not been wearing!

We took the track from *Nadqan* to *Harad* on our return, which shortened the trip considerably. It was a somber group of campers who arrived late that evening in Dhahran. I was lucky to catch the last bus to RT and wasted no time getting into a hot, soapy shower.

Luke went back to find his rig the next weekend, taking with him another axle and several willing friends to help with the recovery. In the few days since we had left the stricken vehicle there had been a windstorm and the Suburban was now almost buried in sand. It was several hours of hard work before they were able to dig it out and fix the axle, before driving back to camp.

19 - PLAYING TRAINS

"WOULD YOU LIKE to explore the *Hijaz* railway this Eid?" Rob asked one day. "It's something I've always wanted to do. I've got photocopied notes on it. Chad Anderson is coming too so there'd be three of us. No need for another vehicle; there are reasonable roads and tracks and there should be the occasional Bedou truck going by."

It sounded like a great idea and I began to research the history of the area. The historic line of the *Hijaz* railway was built by the Turks in the early twentieth century and ran from Turkey to Medina. It was partly destroyed between 1917 and 1918 during the First World War by teams of men under the leadership of an Englishman, T.E. Lawrence. This man sabotaged the railway in an effort to curb Ottoman control in the west of Arabia and became known as 'Lawrence of Arabia'.

Attempts have since been made to reopen the railway. However, although parts of it remained in use for some years, it never fully recovered and today there is little original track on site, on the Arabian side at least.

To make the most of our six days off, we decided to leave as soon after work as possible on our last working day. The day before we left I picked up my *iqama* and company letter granting permission to travel. As I entered the passport office I recognized a young Saudi Arab who had been a patient of mine. He smiled at me.

"Badge number 167543!"

I was astounded.

"How many numbers do you remember?" I asked.

He shrugged.

"Maybe a hundred."

Late that afternoon Chad, Rob and I lurched out onto the highway in Rob's overloaded Land Cruiser. We made good time heading west along the Riyadh expressway, and camped our first night on the plains northwest of the capital. Lights flashed along the horizon as we yanked our cots off the roof rack and crawled into our sleeping bags.

In the morning we were on the road before eight o'clock and an hour and a half later were into the rolling red sands of the *Nafud* desert. By the time we stopped for lunch, the sand had given way to gravel plains and by late afternoon we arrived on the outskirts of *Madina*. A sign directed non-Moslems onto a bypass away from the holy city.

'The railway can be identified by telegraph poles, which still stand beside the remains of the track' read our instructions.

Sure enough, there were the poles. The first station was behind the city wall in *Medina* itself and therefore out of bounds to the likes of infidels such as us, but we backtracked as far as possible to *Muhit*, the second station, just outside the city wall.

Muhit was a surprise—a sophisticated stone structure which had withstood the ravages of time in the desert remarkably well. The station and the fort which had protected it stood at the foot of a hill beneath the remains of an old Arab fort. A plaque over the station entrance proclaimed its name in Arabic script.

We camped in a sheltered area on the hill above the station. Temperatures were remarkably mild for the Saudi Arabian winter. The gibbous moon, between half and full, cast enough light so we could move around without using flashlights, and we savored our solitude so close to the town.

Next morning we again picked up the trail, which was marked by sturdy telegraph poles dated 1907 (some with their cross-pieces still attached). This time we headed north. Scattered villages and farms added a touch of greenery to the sandy expanse, with jagged mountain ridges in the distance.

We wondered how we would manage at the checkpoints, which we had to pass through occasionally along the highways. Chad was married and his wife was listed in his *iqama*, the Saudi Arabian identification document. On the other hand, Rob and I were singles and had our own *iqamas*. I feared that in some of the more conservative areas the authorities would not be pleased with us.

My apprehension was unwarranted, for I never had to show my *iqama* once! The guards at the checkpoints looked at Chad's iqama, assumed I was his wife, and courteously looked no further. This gave rise to many jokes about my wifely obligations to Chad.

It was usually possible to drive along the railway bed, although little of the original rail remained. A narrow dirt track ran alongside the railway and we descended to it whenever the rail bed was unfit to drive on. Beautifully crafted concrete and stone bridges were a testimony to the skill of the European craftsmen who were brought in to do the work so many years ago.

Stations were spaced at an average distance of fourteen miles apart, supposedly to make defense and maintenance easier. All of them were built to the same basic design, though the type of brick varied from place to place. Sometimes yellow brick was used, sometimes reddish or grayish colored stone.

Most of the buildings along the railway had been damaged in an identical fashion: large holes had been dug in the floors, as if someone had been searching for valuables of some kind. In some stations these holes were very deep, probably requiring ropes for the diggers to remove the earth and to get themselves in and out of the pits.

Ueli Bellwader, an archeologist in Jordan, has explained that these holes were not World War I bomb craters but deep holes dug by treasure hunters.

"It may sound crazy," he says, "but people really do believe that the retreating Ottoman soldiers buried gold around the stations. In their frenzy to find it, they have mechanical earth-moving equipment that is demolishing buildings and stretches of the embankment. In Istanbul, maps of the railway are on sale, along with assurances that the crosses marked on the maps note where the Ottoman pots of gold are buried."

There was much rubble and twisted 'I' beam along the track. We 'fingered the thrilling rail,' as did Lawrence back in 1917 and stopped frequently to muse. Here was a piece of rail sticking out of a sand bank, there a whole loco, rusting away under the Arabian sun. A water tank, overturned box cars and scattered pieces of rail—these things we noted as we traveled, anxious not to miss anything of historical significance.

Abu An Na'am was the site of T.E. Lawrence's first attack on the railway. Yellow grass and shrubs surrounded the station, with rugged hills beyond. A snowy owl flew from the water tower as we approached. The station was in fairly good shape and the floor was still partially tiled. I could almost hear a train in the distance.

We occasionally found ourselves stuck in sandy patches and extricated ourselves by pushing, with sand mats under the wheels. The trail was also exceedingly bumpy, and we had to completely repack after each day on the trail. Lids came off bottles, ropes on the roof rack loosened, and plastic bags came untied, the contents distributing themselves randomly about the cabin. Somebody's deodorant stick found its way into the snack box.

At *Hadiyah*, whose small grey fort was trimmed in red stone, many remnants of trains languished, including a complete train on its side. Further up the track, several open graves at *Mudarraj* station held whitening bones and I wondered if those buried there were victims of attacking tribesmen or of cholera, which decimated the Turkish soldiers during those early days.

Jagged mountains began to dominate the skyline as we progressed north. We drove as quickly as possible, pausing only to take photographs of each station as we came to it. As the sun was setting in a blaze of red and gold, we left the highway and made our way into a sandy *wadi,* or dry waterway, for the night. This evening was particularly windy and as careful as we were sand still found its way into the cooking pot.

I poked my head outside the tent the next morning to find the mountains bathed in a delicate golden light. After a hot breakfast of sour-cream pancakes and applesauce we headed off again.

Badayi, the next station, boasted a broken windmill as well as the obligatory fort. Several homes stood nearby, contributing to a large rubbish tip which had grown to surround the historic buildings.

The road became a highway and mountain scenery surrounded us. Still, there was very little traffic to compete with us and we arrived at *Al Ula* earlier than we expected. A small township had grown up around the station, which hid behind the solid steel fences built by the Saudi Arabian Department of Antiquities—it was classed as an historic site and we had no permission to enter!

Outside the gates we contented ourselves by climbing onto an old carriage whose wooden cladding was still largely intact. Slits in the sides of carriages were designed for the gun barrels of the Ottoman soldiers, who protected the trains from the raids of the Bedou.

The railway then crawled amongst rocky outcrops, red spires, and craggy cliffs dotted with green palms, until it reached *Madain Saleh*. The station and several other buildings here have been repaired and restored as a museum and some locos here are in fairly good condition.

Madain Saleh is a famous Nabatean site, dating from the second century BC till the fourth century AD. It is a sister city to Petra, the Nabatean capital, in Jordan. The Nabateans at one time controlled trade and traffic through these parts. They were wealthy and powerful, skilful hydraulic engineers, and charged for protection and water supplies as travelers passed through.

Today little is known of *Madain Salah* except its burial places, with human bones within them. Various sized niches carved inside the tombs accommodated the bodies of children or adults of a family, whereas niches carved on the outsides of family tombs were for illegitimate offspring. Carvings of eagles and lions, amongst other things, decorate the tombs. The details carved into the rock façades are still crisp after centuries of exposure to the elements. Inscriptions on the tombs list who built them, who is buried there and who could use the tombs. There are also warnings and sometimes curses to all who would make inscriptions in a tomb, sell it, rent it or use it for other purposes.

The Nabateans had a sophisticated method of channeling and storing water and there was ample evidence of wells and cisterns. A new study of the whole region was begun in 2001 by French scientists, with aims to investigate and map it out.

We drove around the perimeter fence until we picked up the railway line heading north. It was rough, slow going, on and off the track between steep cliffs. Then the railway climbed up into a high, narrow valley nestled against bulging red cliffs, and for a mile or so it disappeared under a sand drift.

From time to time Rob blew the air horn on the Toyota. It sounded remarkably like a train whistle as we chugged through cuttings or sped along straight sections of the rail bed. Interesting rock formations in the rocky cliffs gave an eerie sense of being on a strange planet, with gnarled forests of stone and twisted peaks.

As we approached *Al Mutalla*, the highest station of the line, a donkey came to the entrance, and then we realized that the whole station was full of animals—goats and sheep. The Bedouin sheep herder came out for a chat and gratefully accepted an orange for his afternoon tea.

Back on the track again we heard a scraping noise, and discovered a fallen shock absorber. A short time later the windscreen wipers spontaneously started up and persisted until Rob removed the fuse. When the track became smoother, we raced alongside the railway across gravel plains until the ruins of an old castle appeared in the distance.

Qalat Al Muazzam stood protected by a strong wire fence, a windmill alongside of it, on one side of the *wadi*. On the other side of the *wadi* stood the station with its fort and water tower. Above the station was another small, ruined fort, the picture presenting a golden panorama in the late afternoon sun.

While making our way across to the station from the castle we made another discovery—a huge square concreted dam, filled with water! We spared no thought before changing into our swimmers and plunging into its coolness. What luck; a bath in the middle of the desert.

A sandy cleft in the hill above the station became our campsite for that evening. It was windy again. I was grateful for the protection in my small tent, for the minimum temperature that night was fifty-two degrees Fahrenheit.

As we progressed north the mountains flattened out, the occasional Bedouin tent nestled alongside a cliff, and herds of camels and sheep wandered freely.

At *Al Asad* station, a single storey barrack building, we surprised a couple of Bedou women in colorful dress as they tended their sheep. They backed off nervously as I got out of the vehicle and spoke to them in Arabic. We exchanged greetings but they refused the oranges I offered and several other women arrived with their herds a few minutes later. We took our photos from inside the station, careful not to frighten or embarrass the women.

Chad's jazz music entertained us on the car stereo system. 'Hi-jazz', we called it. The railway wound down through rocky flats with low reddish-grey hills and clumps of short bushy trees in the *wadis*.

Mid morning we arrived at *Khamisah*, a station built with greenish stone. An interesting walled channel ran behind it, seemingly for water catchment, with storage at the base of the station. The well inside the front door boasted a neat iron framework around it and there were two ovens at the back of the building.

The track led on through a very sandy *wadi*. A local in a pickup was stuck in soft sand near the railway bed, and we were able to help push him out. Shortly afterward we stopped again, this time to admire and photograph a camel in full decorative saddle.

We resumed our journey but suddenly realized that we had lost sight of the railroad. None of us said much although disappointment hung thickly in the air.

It was impossible to turn back as we had to keep moving—the sand was soft and sticky, the *wadi* stretching on as far as the eye could see. And our fuel was running low. Two hours later we still had seen nothing and all but abandoned the search, deciding to go on to the city of *Tabuk* and try again another time. Military signs, "DANGER, DO NOT ENTER," blocked us on each attempt to turn north towards the city.

All of a sudden we spotted the familiar shape of a station on the other side of the valley and made a beeline for it. It was twenty-five miles from the last station we had seen, so we knew we had missed at least one station along the way, as well as the stretch of rail including a tunnel.

This station proved to be one of the three remaining ones along the line, the last one being in *Tabuk* itself and fenced in like the one in *Al Ula*.

The little railway carried bravely on through *Tabuk*, interrupted in parts by roadwork, earthworks, schools, and other buildings. It even became part of a new highway for a few miles before branching off again on its own.

We fuelled up in *Tabuk* mid afternoon and headed homeward, looking for another campsite. Up a dirt track we came to a rough sign: "WARNING—NO ENTERY, EXCEPT MILITANTS." Did we qualify? We decided not, and continued on to pitch our tents in another area, surrounded by low stony *jebels*, rocky outcrops.

Next morning we sped along a modern highway which snaked through jagged red mountains and the occasional village with clusters of date palms. In the city of *Hail* we parked, and stumbled into a real restaurant. Fresh salads, chicken kebabs, and wonderful fresh bread arrived as we relaxed in the family eating area.

Suddenly a man peered around the partition of our cubicle.

"Welcome to Hail," he said. "I saw the Aramco sticker on your car. I also am employed by Aramco."

"Hello, Mr Al Shammari," said Rob.

"How did you know my name?" asked the man, surprised.

"The Al Shammari tribe comes from this area, don't they?" replied Rob with a chuckle. "I had a pretty good chance of being right!"

Our final campsite was on a sandy hillside back in the *Ad Dahna* desert. By the time we chugged through the gates of the compound that afternoon we had driven two and a half thousand miles. Two and a half thousand miles of memories.

20 - GETTING TO THE BOTTOM OF THINGS

DISTURBING REPORTS HAD been coming from women who had taken the shoppers' bus across to Rahima on Tuesday evenings. It seemed that local young boys were ganging up on women and pinching their bottoms, just as they were about to get on the bus.

One morning Pat came in to work nursing a sore back and shoulder.

"A young guy in Rahima kicked me in the back," she said. "Then he hit me on the shoulder. And my back was hurting even before he kicked me!"

Ali, at the Singer Store, was outraged.

"Ah," he said disparagingly, picking his teeth with his Arabian 'toothbrush' stick, "Rahima isn't the same these days. Some of the kids here, they are bad. Three, four times, my shop windows have been broken. I talk to the police but they don't do anything."

I told him about the bottom pinching.

"Is it allowable to do anything to the kids?" I asked. "If we were to catch them would we be in trouble?"

He brightened up.

"Oh that would be very good!" he said. "If you can catch them, take them to the police. The police would be very pleased."

Tuesday evening the shoppers' bus went to Rahima. I was on it. There were a couple of small stones in my pocket, ankle-stingers, nothing that would do any damage. When it was time to go home I had some heavy bags. Perhaps I shouldn't have bought so much, I reflected, but there weren't any young men around tonight anyway, just a couple of little kids playing around the bus. They smiled angelically as I approached the bus. I smiled back and turned to step up. And then came the pinch.

"Right!" I sputtered and jumped down, but the boys were gone.

Should I give up and go home with my bags? Or leave my bags to the mercy of the girls on the bus and run after the boys? Or run after the boys with the bags and find my own way home afterwards?

The two lads were sauntering across the road, snickering between themselves. No woman would risk missing the bus to chase two small boys. Nobody except this little Aussie, I thought, teeth clenched as I strode out, a shopping bag in each hand.

One of the boys glanced casually behind him and a look of horror crossed his face. They started to run again. I threw my two little stones but they went wide. All the way through Rahima I chased those boys, mad at myself for buying so much that evening and weighing myself down. Every so often they looked behind them, only to see me coming after them like a train.

Suddenly, they turned a corner and disappeared. I followed, but the only sign of life there was a man standing in a doorway.

"Did you see two young boys come down this road?" I asked.

"No," he said.

"Well they are bothering the expatriate women and I am angry! This is not good Moslem behavior. They should have respect for women, even women from other countries. If it happens again they will be in big trouble with the police!"

Wondering about my sanity, I walked home. But my efforts paid off. Although I had not been able to catch those two little monkeys and bang their heads together, there were no further attacks in Rahima.

A young hooligan in Al-Khobar did not have such a lucky escape. He chose the wrong woman to hit as he passed by. She was an expert in self-defense, and immediately felled him with a karate chop! It was not an offence for a woman to retaliate if she was attacked, which was a very comforting thing to know. My imagination switched on—maybe I should take classes in martial arts.

Rob and I had become good friends over the previous year, and now he wanted us to commit to each other.

"I am happy with the relationship we have!" I argued. "Let's not get too serious. I don't know that we should. Our backgrounds are quite different and we may not be compatible."

Soon after this charged discussion, Rob struck up a relationship with another girl from Dhahran and I began to feel the pain of separation and more than a little jealousy. He still called me every morning for a while, but I sorely missed the day to day companionship we'd shared. The pain around my heart seemed too much to bear, but I realized I had brought it on myself by pushing Rob away.

New Year's Eve was approaching and Candy and Ian Lyndoch had invited me to a party at their house. Rob was planning to attend also with his new lady. Although I had been the one to put the brakes on our relationship, I was feeling rather low and did not want to see Rob with someone else.

Tanya reminded me that the theme of the party was Middle Eastern.

"Why don't you go as an Arab woman with your face covered?" she said. "Then you won't have to face anyone, but can still attend the party."

The more I thought about it, the more I liked the idea. Without another word I began assembling my costume. I already had the traditional *abaya* and full veil, and a long black scarf. Black stockings and borrowed black leather gloves completed the outfit.

I arrived at Lyndoch's early and entered the house nervously, sliding into the kitchen and leaving a plate of nibbles as my contribution to the party food. Candy caught sight of me and looked startled for a moment. Then she grinned.

"Oh," she said. "You've come as a Saudi woman—great idea! Great costume! Who are you really?"

I suddenly decided to be mute for the evening and pressed a finger to my lips.

"Ahhhh!" she said knowingly. "You don't talk. OK. Have a nice evening!"

At first I was apprehensive but after the first guests arrived the fun began. I realized the transformation an actor must experience while in costume on stage. There was a great deal I could do to entertain people without speaking.

Hugging and kissing each guest in turn was easy, and gradually I took more and more liberties. I ran my black leather fingers teasingly over shoulders, patted guests on heads and hands, and beckoned enticingly. Several times I was asked to dance, and flung myself into the disco with enthusiasm if not grace.

Between dances I sat cross-legged on the sofa and answered questions from other guests with gestures and head movements. They 'discovered' that I was married with five children, lived on camp and that my husband did not know I was at the party.

When Rob arrived, I was in full swing. I stroked his face with my gloved hand, and with remarkable boldness rushed at his lady friend and hugged her enthusiastically. She flinched in surprise.

The veil was oppressive and blinding. I felt a new rush of sympathy for the untold women in this country who had to wear it every day with no relief. It was difficult to keep track of who I had greeted, but I must have caressed one man's shoulder once too often for I was later told that his wife had threatened to "deck" me if I had done it again!

Luckily I overheard a fellow guest when he vowed to unmask me at midnight. Well before twelve o'clock I had vanished from the party and was safely lying in my own bed. For the moment the pain of seeing Rob with another woman was overshadowed by the adrenaline rush of the evening.

Everyone on camp was bursting with curiosity about the identity of the mystery woman, and finally I was asked about it. Without lying I managed to convey the impression that I had not been able to attend the function. After the party, Ian had reportedly said, "I don't know who that woman was, but I hope she comes to our New Year's party next year!"

21 - DIFFERENCES

THERE WERE MANY cultural differences which I needed to get accustomed to.

Ways of communicating: I began one evaluation by asking questions about the patient's symptoms.

"Is your pain worse now than it was before?"

She said nothing but clicked her tongue. I sighed. Why was she upset by the question? This happened frequently in my evaluations and I didn't know what to do about it.

Many of the women had no idea about how their bodies worked or how to cooperate with an exercise program. After all, they had always been taught that their flesh should be hidden away.

I suspected that these Arabian women were fed up with the questions and simply wanted to get on with the treatment. This suspicion was reinforced by a wizened old Bedouin, who loudly proclaimed in Arabic that she had come for a massage, not to be interrogated, and promptly walked out!

I asked Suheim for his opinion of the tongue clicking and he roared with laughter.

"That is their way of saying 'yes' to your question! They are not annoyed at all."

I heaved a sigh of relief.

Indian patients had a habit of wagging the head from side to side in respect, or when the answer was "Yes." My voice would trail off into silence while I became mesmerized by the head wobbling, somehow unable to continue my train of thought. Finally I decided to keep my eyes fixed on the evaluation form while doing the subjective portion, so as not to be distracted.

Generosity: The Saudi Arabian people have to be the most generous people I have ever met. I quickly learned that if I expressed admiration for something, it was bound to be given to me. To avoid embarrassment, I should simply smile and nod and keep my appreciation to myself. Before I learned this however, I was presented with a pair of brightly decorated Saudi Arabian shoes, a bottle of expensive perfume, and several pieces of clothing.

Logic: There is Western logic and there is Eastern logic. And sometimes it seems there is no logic at all. Some expats, perhaps unfairly, called Saudi Arabia the "Logic-free Zone". I believed that if West and East could look at issues from each others' point of view they might be surprised at just how logical they *both* were.

Many people believe that the Almighty has predestined everything to the point where anything that happens occurs because of His will. "*Inshallah*," or "the will of Allah," is probably the best-known Arabic word to an expatriate.

Along part of the seashore on the Ras Tanura compound ran a rock wall, which protected the shoreline against the pounding wave action of the sea. After every storm the wall and the beach path adjoining it needed repair. Over the years the water had eroded the foreshore and threatened the houses on the other side of the beach path. Something had to be done.

Much discussion went on about the feasibility of installing groynes in the bay, to dampen the effects of heavy seas and encourage the growth of protective sandbars. But it was an expensive proposition, and an Arabian maintenance supervisor was once heard to say, "*Inshallah*, everything will be alright. The sea will get tired."

There are those in Western cultures who espouse the same philosophy. Recently I heard of a sailing couple who believed the Almighty would protect them in spite of themselves, to the extent that they had no need to check their holding when they anchored. They ended up on a reef.

'*Inshallah*,' is a fine sentiment. However, the phrase was often used in excuse, for if the speaker didn't do the right thing or suffered as the result of his own foolishness, it must have been the will of God.

I realize that the 'Inshallah mentality,' is *not* intrinsically Islamic and not every Moslem subscribes to it. The prophet Mohammed once rebuked a man for not tying his camel securely and allowing it to escape. The little story is told to emphasize one's responsibilities in life, *as well as* relying on Allah, who has given us brains with which to think.

In the early days of western presence in Kingdom, it was said that car accidents were always blamed on foreigners, for if they were not there the accident would not have happened.

One day an expat from Ras Tanura drove into Rahima where another car rammed into his vehicle, overturning and badly damaging it. The driver of the car was a young boy of eight or ten years of age, who happened to be the son of a *mutawa,* a religious policeman. Fortunately, nobody was injured and the *mutawa* took full responsibility, paying all damages. That, I thought, was real morality.

Traditions: Once a year on the tenth day of the Islamic month of Muharram, the Shiites observe Ashura, the festival of mourning. At this time they remember the grandson of the Prophet Muhammad, Imam Husayn, who was killed in an ambush in 680 AD, along with almost all of his family. A series of elaborate rituals is performed, including self-flagellation, and sometimes at the clinic we saw serious injuries resulting from this.

We had a high percentage of "no shows" from our Shiite patients on this day. They knew they were not going to keep their appointments but permitted us to make them anyway, for their ceremony was not approved of by the Sunni majority, or by Aramco.

After mutilating themselves with whips, sticks, fists, chains and knives, patients would present in emergency with various injuries, even to the extent of fractures. It was a little disturbing to me to see people willing to harm themselves like this, in spite of the prophet Mohammad's injunction, "there shall be no inflicting of harm on oneself."

Language: English truly is a difficult language and being a therapist in Arabia had its moments. I admire all those who master English as a second language. Arabic was also difficult to learn, but it became increasingly important for me to communicate in Arabic for as the company tried to 'Saudiize,' the number of Saudi Arabian patients increased.

One of my back patients was an educated man and I assumed that his English would be better than my Arabic. The evaluation went something like this:

"How did you hurt your back?"

"I don't know."

"Well, then, what were you doing when you first felt the pain?"

"I wasn't doing anything."

"Where *were* you, when you first felt the pain?"

"I was in my house."

"Yes but were you sitting, standing, walking, bending over or lying down when you first felt the pain?"

"I told you, I was doing nothing."

Exasperation rose in my throat and I forced it down with a sigh.

"Let's start again. What *position* was your body in when you first felt the pain come?"

His face lit up. "Oh! What *position* am I in? I am an engineer!"

I asked another patient what kind of work he did.

"I don't do anything!" he replied, affronted. "I'm a supervisor."

Even native Arabic speakers didn't always understand each other. Suheim would help when I needed him but sometimes he would give up, too.

"I don't understand these people," he would complain.

I had to be careful when speaking, that I did not unwittingly cause offence by using wrong words. There is no "p" in the Arabic language so "p" is pronounced "b". "Parking," becomes "barking," and "post office," becomes "bost office." When shopping for a dress zip one day I was advised by an American woman to say "zipper," rather than "zip," as it could be taken as "zib," the Arabic word for a male private part.

Sex discrimination: Before I came to Saudi Arabia, I had heard that the Arabs only want male children and considered girls to be inferior. So, why did fathers carry their little girls around proudly on their shoulders? And why did mothers dress them like princesses and parade them in public?

I never saw any evidence that Saudi Arabs disliked their female children and came to the conclusion that society in Arabia was very much like my own in that regard—yes, fathers were proud to have a male child to carry on their name but girls were also very much loved when they came along.

An Arabian patient told me that he had eight daughters.

"What? No sons?" I asked.

He smiled and shrugged.

"It is from God, what can we do!" he said.

Family size: Saudi Arabs were encouraged by the government to have as many children as possible, to strengthen the nation. I discovered, to my amazement, that one Saudi Arabian woman, at the age of twenty-five, had six children.

"That's nothing," she told me, "my sister has been married for thirteen years and has eighteen children!" None of them were twins.

Cultural mixes: A woman in *abaya* and veil approached our reception desk one day and stood at the window with a referral in her hand. Suheim fired off a couple of rapid questions in Arabic.

"*Huh?*" she said.

We came to know Maggie well. I liked her. She was a young American woman who had married an employee of some prominence in the company and had happily embraced Islam and the Arabic way of life.

She dressed as any Saudi Arabian woman would, in the full veil and *abaya*, but also wore black gloves and black stockings to cover the white skin of her extremities. Her red Mercedes sports car was often seen flying around the camp and it was a miracle she never collided with anything while wearing the veil.

Maggie's initial interaction with Suheim led me to believe that she wasn't very fluent in Arabic, although she used "*Alhumdulillah* (Praise God)," frequently in her conversations. She came in from time to time for treatments for various ailments and I suspected she came for social reasons as much as for treatment.

One day she told us that her husband's son from a previous marriage had come to live with them. The boy was apparently quite unruly and Maggie had difficulty controlling him. I suspected that he had been plucked from his home in the US and his (now probably frantic) American mother. Then the boy went missing from Maggie's home.

He was discovered a week or two later, hiding in an unoccupied house on camp. Boys from his class had been supplying him with food and blankets. I've often wondered if this boy ever adapted to life in Saudi Arabia, or if he was able to return to his life in the US.

Other western women lived as dependent wives of Saudi Arabs on camp. One English girl appeared very happy with her life there, but a Finnish girl admitted that she missed her friends and family back home. It must have been lonely for those without companions from their home countries, although living on the compound was a lot easier than in the community outside.

Marriage: Moslems are permitted to have up to four wives at a time, and many of my patients had more than one wife. One young man, who came for treatment of back pain, had something important on his mind.

"I have four wives," he began uneasily, "and every night I am busy. *Very* busy. Do you understand?"

I nodded, wondering where this would lead.

"Is this bad for my back, when I am very busy like this?"

"This kind of exercise is usually good for your back," I said. "Tell me, when you are 'very busy,' and immediately afterwards, do you have any back pain?"

He considered for a moment and then decided he did not.

"Well then," I said brightly, "You don't need to worry. This kind of activity is not going to hurt you. It might even be good for you!"

His face lit up.

"Thank you! Thank you very much! Because every night I am very busy."

Heredity: Sickle cell anemia is a disease which afflicts many in Saudi Arabia. It is more prevalent in the dark races, particularly from Africa. Sufferers can experience severe pain from an early age as their red blood cells adopt a flattened appearance ('sickle-cell') which limits the oxygen-carrying ability. It is devastating as joints, particularly hip joints, deteriorate.

One young lady I saw from time to time as a patient was only twelve years of age, and already hobbled around like an old woman. Her hip joints were too fragile to bear her weight without excruciating pain.

The youngest patient I ever saw with bilateral hip replacements was a Saudi Arab aged twenty-one. It is a tragedy which could so easily be averted by prohibiting marriage between first cousins. Some Saudi Arabs have made the decision to choose spouses from other tribes but unfortunately many still prefer to marry within their families, perpetuating this disease.

Hygiene: Westerners often chuckled about Eastern toilets—those holes in the floor which the locals squatted over when answering calls of nature. Our toilets were certainly better, more sophisticated.

A popular diagram replicated in the bathrooms of many expatriate homes sported a figure squatting on a pedestal. The diagram had a cross over it. Beside this diagram was another figure sitting on a pedestal. This diagram had a tick over it. The humor was obvious—the quaint custom of squatting on the toilet seat was not to be tolerated here.

One day, while reading a Physical Therapy journal, I came across an article on the physiology of defecation and why the Eastern posture was the best position for this activity. There was even an adaptive device available which fit over a Western toilet so one could squat on it.

"Wow, look at this!" I exclaimed to Suheim.

He was just as fascinated as I was. Sometimes we Westerners are not as smart as we think we are.

Social: There are many other differences between West and East. I noticed that there were no old folks' homes or hospices in Saudi Arabia, for needy people are absorbed into the extended family and nurtured with love.

Children generally take their obligations towards their parents seriously and treat them with respect. If someone is in need and has nobody to help, they can call for alms from anybody in the community, or approach a prince who is always willing to listen and reach into his pocket. I decided there was much to learn from the Saudi Arabian way of life.

On the other hand, the eldest son in a Saudi Arabian family has so many demands from female members of his household that there is little time for himself. He is expected to chauffeur them all wherever they want to go—and he is forever apologizing to his supervisor at work for taking time off.

The Calendar: The *Hijri* calendar, used in Saudi Arabia, is a lunar calendar, with twelve lunar months and three hundred and fifty-four or fifty-five days in the year. It is not synchronized to the seasons and there is a drift of eleven or twelve days annually. The first year was the year in which the Prophet Mohammed emigrated from Mecca to Medina. This calendar is used by Moslems to plan their religious festivals.

Especially in the early days of Aramco, patients were sometimes flown to the USA for specialist treatment. It was amusing to imagine the consternation of the medical staff when they looked at the patient's file and saw his or her birth date. It could read something like 1364!

22 - ON BEING STRUNG ALONG

TANYA AND I SIGNED up to do a rappelling course under the instruction of an American in Dhahran. Ted was very good at everything he did. With great empathy and lashings of humor he nurtured each one in the class until we had mastered every skill. He gave us confidence in his rope and tackle and taught us how to check and double-check every application before trusting our lives to it. It was a far cry from my first rappelling experience with a rope harness on a cliff face in Ma'aqala.

In spite of a healthy fear of heights I soon found myself enjoying this sport and it was handy on the caving trips we sometimes embarked upon. I was able to cope with some very high cliffs after a short time.

The equipment Ted used was the best and he kept it always in prime condition. Whenever possible I joined scout training expeditions as an instructor, in the escarpments around Riyadh and in the Asir, the mountain range in the west of the country.

One of the highest airstrips in the world is located in the Asir, and Aramco scout leaders struck a deal with the company. The yearly scout camp not only provided the scouts with rappel training, but also provided high altitude landing and take-off experience for Aramco pilots. The flights were free for the boys and for us, their trainers, and although we worked hard for the week of the camp we wouldn't have missed it for the world.

We arrived at the camp a day or so earlier than the boys, to set up the rappel sites in advance. Carrying bags of supplies up the hill from the base camp on the first day seemed strangely difficult until we remembered that we were accustomed to working at sea level, not at ten thousand feet.

The rappel sites were of varying difficulties, and there was also a traverse, set up with ropes and back-up lines, across a deep ravine. It struck terror into the hearts of most would-be riders. Almost everyone, adult or child, hesitated a long time before stepping out into the void, and many chickened out altogether. I had one session operating the traverse. It gave me great satisfaction to be able to persuade a reluctant child to trust the ride. Moans and screams of terror turned into yells of delight and most riders came back for more.

Not only was I fastened to the traverse setup, but to a sturdy tree by a line from a carabiner at the back of my waist belt. As the thrill seeker flew across the gully, I would release a lever which activated the brake, to pull him up short. He would dangle crazily, certain that he was about to plunge into the abyss, while friends laughed and took photographs to amaze the folks at home.

Occasionally one of the adults took a turn riding the traverse. The first man to try it on my shift cautiously released his footing on terra firma and began the downward hurtle. At the appropriate instant I released the handgrip to pause his descent and suddenly my world turned upside down. I had been flipped forward, with only my tether to the tree restraining me from plunging into nothingness. Flat on my belly, I peered wonderingly over the edge of the ravine.

Several people who had witnessed the incident began to shout. The first to my rescue was Richard, the Scout master in charge.

"Stay very still. Don't worry, we'll get you out of there in no time." He spoke quietly and reassuringly although in truth I felt more surprised than fearful. I was certainly going nowhere!

Before anything else though, I had to release the poor man dangling in mid-air. Gently I squeezed the handgrip and sent him merrily on his way to the other side. Then Richard pulled me carefully to my feet.

It was a matter of simple physics really—the rope attached to the tree, from the connection at the back of my harness, was at a slight angle from the traverse lines. The man on the traverse was heavier than I, and when I stopped his flight, his weight jerked the line straight and pulled me sideways with it. There had never been any real danger; Ted's expertise with knots and lines had seen to that. It was 'just one of those things' that adds to the bank of experience.

It took us so long to set up the traverse at the beginning of the week that we were loath to break it down every day, so some of us volunteered to camp at the top of the slope, having no scout-minding duties. Our presence would deter any would-be thieves who might be lurking.

We enjoyed the tranquility of the mountains, after the boys had left in the afternoons, and the stupendous views from the top in the mornings. A troop of baboons cavorted about not far from the rappelling area but they never bothered us. Around sunrise and sunset they became active, squabbling and squalling among the bushes of the escarpment and bounding up and down the faces of the cliffs where they lived.

Small cedars grew around the edges of the track and someone decided that since Juniper berries were used to flavor gin, alcohol flavored by cedar berries must be 'sin'!

One day, up on a trail that wound close to our campsite, we were stunned to see two old Japanese ladies twirling their parasols. They were guests at a magnificent hotel on an adjacent hillside. Tourism, albeit limited, had arrived in Saudi Arabia.

At the end of the week, it was time to return to the Eastern Province. At the airport security check-in, a small Swiss army knife in my pocket set off alarm bells. The blade was about an inch long. Prior to the terror attacks of 2001, small knives were still permitted on airlines and I always kept this knife with me. I was beckoned aside into a special room, where two female Arabian security officers found it and wanted to confiscate it.

"*Laa! Laa!* No! No!" I said, shaking my head vigorously.

They paused, confused. Then they suggested breaking off the blade.

"No! Don't do that either," I pleaded.

Finally they adjusted their veils and escorted me outside to speak to the man in charge. He took one look at the small knife and dismissed the case with a wave of the hand and a rolling of eyes. I escaped, tucking my treasure securely back into my pocket.

Outside, we realized that Lynn, Richard's wife, had not made it through.

"What could be the matter?" Richard worried.

Finally Lynn burst out of the customs area, flustered but relieved.

"They were convinced I had drugs in my handbag," she said. "I've never been so scared in my life—I had such trouble convincing them that it was only a packet of instant oatmeal!"

23 - TYING THE KNOT, SUNNI STYLE

"MY PARENTS WANT ME to get married," Suheim had told me. He'd dallied for a long time but finally decided that he was ready and his mother leapt into action.

It is the custom in Saudi Arabia for the female elders of the family to advise on the girl, as after all they are the only ones who have the freedom to see behind the veil. The males at the head of the household have the final say and make the arrangements.

So it was that one of Suheim's female cousins suggested a young lady from a good family in Dammam and the wheels began to turn. The chosen one was working as a ward clerk in the Aramco clinic in Dhahran.

"Please, please!" Suheim begged me, "The next time you go to Dhahran, go and see her and tell me what you think of her!"

"How can I give you advice?" I asked. "My opinion may be very different from yours!"

"No, really," he urged, "I just want to know what you think of her."

I didn't know my way around the hospital in Dhahran, so Maria arranged for one of the other therapists to show me around as if I were a new therapist. My encounter with Jowahir was brief.

"Hello," I said and she smiled, returned the greeting and turned away.

Green eyes, fair skin, nice smile. She was slender, dressed very liberally for a Saudi Arabian woman—like the Palestinian and Syrian Moslems in a white, flowing gown with a white scarf covering her hair but not her face. Suheim plied me with questions afterwards.

"Is she pretty? Tell me!"

"Well, I thought she was nice," I said, and described the young lady as I remembered her.

"Oh good," he said, pleased. "But is she pretty?"

"Well, I think so, but you might not!"

When the day arrived for his first interview with Jowahir's father, he was very nervous. His own father accompanied him. Jowahir's father was congenial. They enjoyed a long visit and then, "I can't believe it!" Suheim told me. "He brought Jowahir in with no head covering! I got to see her uncovered at the very first visit!"

Suheim sweated for several weeks before Jowahir's family accepted his proposal. He knew that during this period they were busy collecting data on him and sending out spies to check on his behavior.

The engagement lasted over three months.

"You may visit Jowahir at any time," her father said. "But you are never to take her out of the house. And the doors must be open to others of the family while you are visiting."

Jowahir was apparently very shy, although those who knew her at work reported that she thought the sun, moon and stars shone out of Suheim. She would sit and listen while Suheim talked, and he was very good at talking.

As the weeks passed, Suheim discussed the impending marriage with Pat and me. He was not really in love, he realized, but love would probably come after the wedding. And the wedding would happen—for if he didn't want to go ahead with it, there would be massive embarrassment and loss of face for both families.

The wedding night arrived and I was interested to see how the celebration would compare with the Shiite wedding I had attended. Pat and I sat together in the wedding hall. We had some inkling of what lay ahead, as Suheim's family was responsible for the reception and the cost of the wedding was exhorbitant.

The hall was tastefully, even extravagantly, decked out in white and gold. As the female guests arrived, they began to dance to sophisticated music. Once again there was a female band but there was an order and grace about the proceedings.

At the next table from us, a woman stood and danced slowly and sensually for her tablemates. She cut a perfect figure in an exquisite black gown. Her thick wavy hair framed a fair-skinned face, with fine features and flashing green eyes. I could imagine her as a descendent of the Queen of Sheba.

When it came time for the newlyweds to appear before the crowd, I looked for Suheim. He would be terrified—he had told me so.

"You have no idea!" he had exclaimed. "The whole hall will be full of women and these women, all of them, are going to be looking at me. Whatever I do will be the wrong thing. If I look at Jowahir they'll say I can hardly wait to get my hands on her. If I look around, they'll say I have a wandering eye. If I smile or if I don't, I'll still be in trouble."

Suheim did look slightly nervous when he entered, but he carried himself magnificently. Over his *thowb* he wore a robe of black with gold edging and looked quite regal.

With his eyes downcast and with just the hint of a smile, he accompanied his lovely bride, who shimmered in ivory beaded silk, up the aisle.

After they left the hall, Pat and I slipped out to congratulate them and took some photographs before returning to the reception. The buffet tables strained under a banquet hard to match anywhere and the guests lined up in orderly fashion to fill their plates.

When he returned to work after the honeymoon, Suheim was a different person. He was now the head of a household, a husband and potential father. Life was more serious; religion became suddenly important to him. He took time off at prayer times now, to go to the mosque, and more fervently lobbied for a transfer to Dhahran clinic. Marriage changed everything.

24 - RED SAILS IN THE SUNSET

ROB HAD BROKEN off with his girlfriend from Dhahran and, although there was an uneasiness about our friendship, once again we two were enjoying weekends together. In the summer of 1994 we completed a sailing course with Jim Manly of the yacht club, and Rob bought his own boat, a sixteen foot Hobie cat called the 'Golden Eagle'.

She had bright yellow hulls, and orange and red sails. She did fly, but not very fast, and we were towed in by the rescue crew many times that year. There were always repairs to make and we came last in all the races at the yacht club.

On one magnificent day in the Persian Gulf, blue water curled about us in fifteen knots of wind. We were flying along on the "Golden Eagle", Rob on the tiller and me hanging out on the trapeze, when there was a strange sound like cardboard tearing and my trapeze harness suddenly slackened.

Frantically I looked about for the cause.

"The boat's coming apart!" I yelled.

"Be more specific!" Rob yelled back.

The little boat was indeed coming apart—the upper part of the starboard hull had stripped right off the pontoon, pulled up by the starboard stay for the mast. The mast began to tilt alarmingly to port and soon the rescue boat was on its way out to us.

The boat was old and heavy. On a couple of occasions we almost sank her, simply by forgetting to put the plugs in the drain holes! Luckily the water in the Gulf was warm and there was no personal harm in being immersed on a regular basis.

As part of our course we had learned the 'man overboard' drill. One day as we coasted towards the beach after a day on the bay, Rob said suddenly, "Are you comfortable?"

"Yes," I said, mystified, and without another word he rolled off the boat and into the water.

"Darn you!" I yelled.

I knew what to do, but doing it alone was more than I could manage. With one foot tethering the jib sheet, my hands sheeting in the main and a knee to steady the tiller, I tried desperately to go through the 'man overboard' procedure. *Bear away...jibe...swing into the wind...stop just downwind of the person in the water.* Three times I tried but didn't manage the maneuver to Rob's satisfaction so he refused to climb aboard. Shaking with exhaustion, I turned the little craft and sailed away.

"She's leaving him there!" hooted someone on shore, but I only needed a few minutes of rest and a fresh approach.

A few minutes later I had the energy to try again and this time Rob accepted my efforts.

"I wanted to know if you could save me if I fell in," he said with a grin.

The Ras Tanura yacht club was a short drive from the border of the residential camp. Only members could use the facilities. On sunny summer weekends the club became a bustling centre of activity.

Windsurfers and sailboats flew about the bay, people sunbathed, and an Indian chef served meals from the kitchen, including grilled *hamour,* grouper, to die for. During the week the clubhouse was usually deserted and the boats sat on blocks in rows in the yard behind the building.

Race days were exciting. There were usually three races, and two boat classes—up to six Hobie Cats and a fleet of Lasers. Each participant received a T-shirt to remember the event by. Some of the non-racing wives kept time, rang bells and raised flags, amid great hilarity.

After the races a sponsor such as Hempel Paints would present trophies and prizes. At Christmas time and on other special occasions we signed up for dinners at the yacht club and, some toting non-descript bottles in brown paper bags, arrived en masse for a jolly evening out. There was something magical about the plain little building on the waterfront, with the marvelous sandy beach in front and the desert behind.

Boat owners were bound by strict regulations. You could only go out for the day if you went to the Coast Guard station and signed out your boat. At the end of the day you would take your boat out of the water, park it up on blocks, and sign in again with the

Coast Guard. There were strict limits as to where you could sail, and you must never land on the residential beach. One day, at the helm of the Hobie, I strayed a little too far north. Swiftly the Coast Guard boat zoomed out toward us, and we tacked south to avoid a confrontation.

Every boat was required to be registered and had a number. Even windsurfers needed a registration number. Photographs were essential for your boat registration, with you in the picture and the number visible on your boat. Friends with windsurfers would stick temporary numbers on their boards for the photographs and remove them afterwards.

One employee, seriously training for swim marathons, had been discovered by a very perturbed coast guard several kilometers out from shore. An enquiry was launched and much discussion resulted. The conclusion was that the swimmer could be permitted to continue training. However, he would have to register himself with a hull number!

25 - BAD APPLES

"HELP! HELP!" SHE screamed. Everyone in the commissary—the young men at the check-outs, the shoppers in the aisles, the manager in his office—looked up, startled. The young Filipina woman who had been waiting by the entrance shouted her story of betrayal.

Cecilia was a housemaid, who worked for a Saudi Arab doctor and his family on camp. Now her contract was up and she was being taken to the airport. Filipina girls would typically come out on two-year contracts, after which they would return home.

The doctor had stopped to pick up a few things at the commissary before he drove Cecilia through the gates for the last time, and while the girl was waiting for him she saw her only chance for justice. At the top of her voice she told the story of not having been paid by the doctor for the entire time she had been working for him and his family.

The manager of the commissary leaped from his desk. He ushered Cecilia and the doctor into his office and immediately called Personnel to sort out the mess. I don't know if Cecilia was finally paid the salary due her, but I do know that others in her position have been in the same situation, leaving the country with nothing but tears to show for their long and often arduous duties in Kingdom. Every country has its bad apples, and Saudi Arabia is no different.

One day a teacher at the school for expatriate children discovered a Pakistani cleaner asleep in a cupboard. The man told the teacher he was tired because he had not been paid for months and had no money to buy food. He was lucky to have been discovered; the teacher took him and his co-workers to town and bought them enough food to keep them going until he had reported their case to Aramco and the contracting company was made to pay up.

On another occasion twenty-two Nepalese workers were found crammed into a tiny room in Al Khobar. They had not been paid, and had been beaten as well. They owned only the clothes they stood up in and their employer still held their passports so they couldn't leave the country.

Two expatriates from our compound 'raised Cain' until they got the Labor Court on the case and got together enough in donations to provide food and clothing and pay for their flights home. The employer was ordered to pay damages and return the men's passports, but at the last moment he told the court that he was not actually in charge of the workers—his wife was!

Proceedings had to begin again. Sadly, these men went home without the pay due them, but at least they got to go home. I wondered how many others had been in the same position with nobody to fight for them, and what their end had been.

I could never understand why expatriates were involved in crimes within Kingdom, as the penalties under Sharia law included beheading, lashes and amputation of extremities. In the December of 1996, two British nurses, employed at the King Fahad Military Medical Center in Dhahran, were arrested for the murder by stabbing of an Australian nurse. Her body had been found in the nurses' residence there and the two British nurses had been picked up after video surveillance cameras showed them using her credit cards at the automated teller machine in the Bank.

The British nurses were incarcerated in the Dammam Central Prison until May 1998. One of them had faced beheading and the other eight years in prison plus five hundred lashes (which were never given). Under Saudi Arabian law, a murder victim's closest relatives can waive the execution order and accept 'blood money,' in lieu. The nurses were granted a pardon by the King after the victim's brother in Australia agreed to accept one million and seven hundred thousand Australian dollars 'blood money.'

The Industrial Training Centre (ITC) ran classes for young Saudi Arabs on camp. There was occasionally ill-feeling between young men from different tribes and sometimes this led to direct conflict. One day a knock came at the door and one young Arab said insolently to another, "Open the door, you Indian!"

This was the ultimate insult, for Indians performed the menial tasks within the Kingdom. The incident resulted in a fight outside after class and during this fight one young lad was killed by a knife.

The killer was, of course, sentenced to death by beheading.

In spite of these incidents, there was such a slight risk of criminal activity that I felt safer in Saudi Arabia than anywhere else I'd ever been. I walked everywhere at will with no fear of molestation.

Instances of cruelty were unusual in the local community and for the most part I found Saudi Arabs to be generous, kind and hospitable. Saudi Arabian men would step away from queues in banks and shops to let me go first, bring gifts to me at the clinic and offer me assistance of any kind if ever I was in need.

I planned at one time to buy my father a complete Saudi Arabian outfit—the *thowb* (white robe), *ghutra* (head scarf), *agal* (black 'rope' over the headdress) and *taghea* (skullcap) as well as sandals. I spoke to a Saudi Arabian patient of my plans, and the next time he came for treatment he brought a package with the things I had been speaking of!

"You didn't need to do that," I scolded gently. "That was most generous of you!"

He shook his head with a shy smile. "We must look after the old people."

26 - LAW AND ORDER

MY FRIEND THE bank manager, Abdul Al Mota, continued to come to my house weekly for several months, missing few sessions of conversational English. He invited me to his home for a meal, and I met his wife and two beautiful children.

Abdullah was besotted with his family and gave me photographs of the children and a travel video of his favorite haunts. Among several other gifts, he gave me a Quran and reading material about Islam. Abdul must have had connections in high places for he told me that if ever I was in trouble I should contact him and he would be able to help.

One evening he gave me another gift—a stuffed turtle. My mind raced wildly, thinking of possible ways to reject it without hurting his feelings.

"Oh, Abdul," I exclaimed, "That is so thoughtful of you! I can't accept this; it must be very precious to you."

"That's alright," he said. "Take it. My family doesn't like it!"

How could I tell him that I also did not like the turtle? I graciously accepted the gift, and thrust it into the back of my wardrobe out of sight. Years later I left it with the Ras Tanura Theatre Group in their prop cupboard. Australian customs officials would never have allowed it into the country anyway.

Time passed and one day I realized I hadn't heard from Abdul for several months. Enquiries uncovered the sad truth. Abdul and his family had fled the country, never to return. He had been caught borrowing funds from customers' accounts to invest in the stock market, and if he had stayed he would most likely suffered the amputation of his right hand.

He had chosen infrequently used accounts to minimize the risk of discovery, and I am quite sure that he fully intended to pay back whatever he borrowed with interest. However one day an Arabian woman tried to withdraw money from her account and discovered that there was nothing in it!

Abdul had made the decision to leave Saudi Arabia immediately, before the investigation was completed, as he knew full well what Sharia law would demand. Even his high connections could not have saved him.

What is even more shocking is the fact that it was the *third time* he had been caught with his hands in the till. It is hard to imagine why the bank allowed him to continue as manager after the first time, let alone the second. I hope Abdul is living a happy life—and an honest one—in exile with his family.

Sharia law can be swift and harsh in Saudi Arabia. You may lose your head for drug smuggling or murder, your right hand for recurrent theft, or be stoned for adultery. There are whippings for other offences.

Every Friday, executions, beatings and amputations are held in public places, and lists of offenders and their punishments are published in the Arab News. The "Green Truth," some called it. I did wonder, however, about the man who was caught smuggling drugs 'by hiding them in his womb'.

In some areas expats were jostled to the front line when an execution was going on, to see what real justice was. Fortunately I never saw an execution although I have read accounts of them. If I ever had the misfortune to be executed by beheading I would pray for a quick, strong executioner with a very sharp sword.

Each year around the holy month of Ramadan the King has the power to issue pardons. It is not uncommon for several hundred pardons to be issued at one time, permitting criminals with major offences to walk absolutely free. In one instance I heard that an expatriate was shot several times in the chest by a disgruntled subordinate—he did not die so it was *only* an attempted murder. The assailant, who gave himself up to police, walked free with a pardon some six to twelve months later.

One Thursday I went with friends to the Qatif market. We arrived mid-morning and I soaked up the sensations—the din of the animal market, the perfume of fruit and vegetables, the textures of mats and baskets, and the wonderful aromas of all kinds of spices in bins. There were a lot of police around but it wasn't until we had returned to camp that we discovered someone had been beheaded in Qatif just before we'd arrived.

My stomach squirmed when I realized that if we'd been a bit earlier we would probably have witnessed it. Executions are usually held on a Friday, the holy day, to give the victim a chance at Paradise, but there was apparently no chance at Paradise for this soul.

Years later I was treating my last patient of the morning when he began to say some vitriolic things about mutawas.

"Hush!" I said frantically. "You could get into big trouble if you start talking like that!"

Fortunately there was nobody else in the department as Mahmoud began to tell me a story through clenched teeth. The execution of his friend in Qatif was the execution I had narrowly missed witnessing. Mahmoud had been in the USA at the time, and had only heard about the event later. His words dripped bitterness.

"My friend refused to close his shop during prayer time. He told the mutawas that the people serving in the shop and the people buying from the shop were not Muslims so why should he close the shop? There were many words between him and the mutawas and finally they dragged him away. His mother was screaming, holding onto his legs while they dragged him. It was terrible. They called him an infidel and so they beheaded him on a Thursday."

One mutawa, a patient told me, had repeatedly harangued local men for not going into the mosque at prayer times. Two of his victims went on holiday to India, and great was their surprise to see this very same mutawa walking the streets there—with a woman on each arm! The men waited for an opportune moment to waylay him and give him a sound beating before they returned to Saudi Arabia. This mutawa gave them no further problems.

An American patient told me of her shopping trip to Khobar on a Thursday. As she and a friend descended from the shoppers' bus, they found crowds and police everywhere and were advised to head for the other side of Khobar. An execution was scheduled in the square near the Shula Mall. Quickly the women disappeared before they were seen by the mob and pushed to the front of the crowd. After it was all over, they ventured back into town. Stunned Indian shopkeepers who had gone to view the execution straggled back to work muttering, "Bad! Bad!"

I asked what the prisoner had done to deserve a Thursday execution. Apparently he had sexually assaulted a two year old child then had drowned him in a pool of water before running him over with a car.

I hoped that the law had convicted the right man. In the Guardian newspaper, an article on capital punishment told of a Sudinese man on death's row in Riyadh for committing a murder, although his passport gave evidence that he'd been out of the country at the time the offence was committed.

During the Gulf War in 1991 there were apparently some difficulties between US marines and mutawas. The religious men objected to the females driving vehicles, flying planes, and wearing masculine clothes. The story is told of a big, black female marine who listened to a tirade from a little mutawa for some time before grabbing him up by the arms and kissing him on the lips! He shot away like a frightened rabbit.

Many of the mutawas were finally moved out of the Eastern Province for the duration of the war, as they were interfering with the war effort. In 1993 they began to drift back again and there were a number of incidents, some provoked by the foolish actions of westerners.

One Aramco woman, dressed provocatively in short sleeves and a skirt above the knees, went to Khobar on the shoppers' bus. Mutawas stormed onto the bus, took the license off the Filipino driver and virtually stranded the passengers for several hours until Aramco officials arrived to sort out the mess.

Some shocking crimes have been committed in Saudi Arabia in spite of the death penalty. In 2002 many expatriates left the country because of terrorist attacks and gruesome killings. However, compared with the crimes committed in Western nations, it still seemed a much safer place to be. Expatriates from all over the world have lived happily in Saudi Arabia for their whole working lives, and many of these would choose to retire here if it were possible.

Friends once crossed the border from Jordan into Saudi Arabia at *Hajj* time, when the border was most crowded. The husband cautioned his wife to be patient as it seemed the wait for processing could be many hours. They were noticed by the Saudi Arab supervisor, who asked to inspect their vehicle, and within thirty minutes they were given the green light to leave.

The husband thanked the supervisor for his assistance and shook his hand. The supervisor said,

"*Afwan*, you're welcome. Your wife, she should not have to wait with all these men."

27 - SHOWCASE IN THE DESERT

I PAUSED IN the mouth of the cavern. Was I totally crazy? Warm, moist air flowed up from underneath me, and I could see only blackness below the damp rock I was standing on. My only motivation to continue was the expectation of my friends above, smiling encouragement and urging me onwards. I suddenly wished I were not the lightest one of the group!

Rob and I were back in our favorite camping area near Ma'aqala, hunting for new *dahls*, or caves. Salim, Rob's work colleague, had enjoyed his caving experience at Wadi Sabsab so much that we had invited him to come again and he accepted happily.

However, after we picked him up he sadly told us that he could not go into any more caves. He had shown his mother the photos taken in Wadi Sabsab and she refused to let him come with us again unless he promised not to do it again. Ever the dutiful son, he would keep that promise.

Our friends Dani and Brian, from Dhahran, were with us on this expedition and we had also invited my new boss, Mary, to come with us in Rob's vehicle. James had resigned and gone back to the USA, and Mary had come to take his position. James had been a workaholic, whereas Mary refused to let work rule her life and took her weekend recreation seriously.

She and Rob were taking a shortcut across a rough area of rocky hillocks on the first afternoon to retrieve a flashlight that someone had left behind, when she spotted a ring of bright green moss around a wide hole.

Hot air flowing out of the cavern was met by cold winter air from outside, creating a moist environment—perfect for moss to flourish. It was right on sunset. Rob stopped briefly to take a GPS reading and then hastened back to camp before darkness descended.

Our first thought on the following morning was to check out the new *dahl* and I, being the lightest one of the group with rappelling experience, was nominated to go in first. I turned on my headlight as I clambered down over black, slippery rocks, asking for more rope on the belay as the entrance curved around a little.

I soon realized that it was possible to scramble down backwards without the rope and called for the others to follow. Twenty feet below the surface and around a bend lurked a wonderful surprise—a large clump of magnificent stalactites. We had finally discovered a real cave! A few yards away the low ceiling opened up into a large room, with prolific formations.

The Great Room, as we called it, boasted a very long, fragile looking 'rope' among a cluster of other stalactites. On another wall hung a long series of 'organ pipes', row upon row. We gasped in wonder. This was much more than we had hoped for. The light from our headlamps revealed formations almost everywhere, and it was a long time before we could bring ourselves to move on.

Hunting around, we found another room behind the organ pipes. Delicate structures clamored for our attention from every direction. We could hardly bear to leave—but duty called. There was work to face on the following day, and it was a long drive home.

We all sensed Salim's disappointment in not being able to explore the cave with us and before we left the area, Rob wanted to give the young man something to remember. At the sheer rock wall where Tanya and I had made our first descent three years previously, Rob set up the ropes and harnesses, a real professional operation this time.

He belayed two of us down before calling on Salim. Salim listened carefully as Rob instructed him on how to position himself and how to let the rope slide through his descender, and he obeyed to the letter.

"I have never seen this done before," he said afterward, "But I knew I would be OK if I did exactly what Rob told me."

I gave Salim the photos I'd taken of his descent.

"I will not show my mother any of these pictures," he said with a gleam in his eye. "Or she would forbid me to do this, also!"

Six weeks went by slowly, each with commitments that held us in camp. We grasped the first opportunity to return to our natural wonderland. Even with the GPS point to aim for, we had to hunt around a bit for the *dahl* entrance as it was so well concealed.

Once again we found our way into the Great Room. Now we had more time to explore. But what lay beyond? Sharp projections of rock protruded into the next opening. This was not going to be a piece of cake. Should we go head first or feet first?

One by one, grunting and exclaiming, spiraling amongst stalactites, rocks and sand, we squeezed through the gap and into the next room. Here under a rock shelf many tiny white projections grew like plant roots. I couldn't resist touching them with the tip of my little finger, and half a dozen little crystals fell into my hand.

"Look out, here comes Attila the Nun!" someone joked.

Gnarled outcrops of rocks, rich red tones in the rocky roof, fragile curling strands of gypsum—there was so much of interest here. Unusual shapes emerged in the torch light and, like cloud watching, it was fun to imagine all kinds of representations. Here was a giant stork, there a snowy white tulip, then the head and neck of a cobra which waited to be charmed out of its basket. Down where the stalactites met the sand, they were encrusted in large, clear crystals. Fallen stalactites and crystals lay amongst it all, matter that had fallen from the ceilings over eons.

We began laying line down as a guide, in case we became disoriented. Each of us carried two sources of light and spare batteries. It was obvious that nobody had ever been into this cave before us because of its pristine condition. Its many delicate formations would surely have been damaged otherwise. With limited space to crawl in, we caused some damage at times. The floor of the cave was mostly twisted and rocky, and we had to be careful not to drop anything which could disappear down a crevice, or to twist an ankle.

There was life within the cave. On our second visit we noticed many small droppings in the sand on the cave floor. Then a slender black shadow shot across in front of me, while two more fluttered around one of the larger rooms. They were moving too fast to define details, but we realized that they were small bats. It was a challenge to try to capture them on film.

They were tiny, grey and birdlike, their wings translucent against the light. Around dusk they could be seen swooping around inside the mouth of the cave, faster and faster, their numbers increasing, until by twos and threes they spun out into the darkness.

There were other caves in the *Ma'aqala* area. Since finding 'our' *dahl* we became aware of other major caves. Some were much larger and each had its own points of interest, although the 'Mossy Dahl,' as we first called it, appeared to rival the others for the extent of its formations. Nearby we found a smaller cave, which was alive with bats and which we called 'Cave of a Thousand Wings'.

We managed to connect with John Pint, another cave enthusiast, and took him to see our find. He reciprocated by showing us several other caves which he had surveyed. John, who was in Kingdom as a schoolteacher, was later given a government appointment to explore caves and write reports on them.

There was often a rush of air in or out of the openings of the bigger dahls. At first we were mystified by the phenomenon of cold air coming out of an opening in summer time and hot air coming out in the winter time. The truth is that the temperature in a large *dahl* is a constant ambient temperature, apparently cool in summer and warm in winter. The temperature in the Mossy Dahl was a steady eighty degrees Fahrenheit, warm enough to make us sweaty as we worked ourselves through the passages below.

The weather in this area is capricious. There are often pressure changes in the atmosphere and short, violent rain storms pass through frequently. When a band of low pressure goes across an area, the large volume of air within an extensive cave complex is then at relatively higher pressure and rushes out of the small opening. It takes some time to equalize the pressure, and by then another front has passed through, meaning that there is almost always a flow of air along the cave system.

Caves are usually named in the language of the country that they are found in, so our "Mossy Dahl" was duly named "*Dahl Tuhlub*". It remains one of the highlights of my camping days in Arabia.

28 - A WOMAN'S PLACE

SUHEIM BELIEVED HE was 'out of sight and out of mind,' in Ras Tanura, and that if he could only get to work in the Dhahran clinic his chances of getting company sponsorship to the USA for training would be much greater. He suspected that I was holding him back professionally, blocking his transfer because I wanted to keep him in Ras Tanura. I assured him I was not, and that if he wanted a transfer I would not prevent it.

Suheim's capabilities as receptionist and physical therapy assistant were exceptional. He had a wonderful way with people and could almost always send an upset patient away smiling. His English language was almost perfect; he could fool anybody on the telephone into thinking that he was American. In fact he was convinced that expats got better service in some areas, and so always used his 'American' voice if he wanted snappy results!

Suheim finally got his transfer but unfortunately was never sponsored to study for a degree. I felt somehow that he had missed his calling.

Perhaps a friend was right when he said that Suheim should have been picked up in Personnel. With his excellent people skills he would have been an asset to that department. He later got a job in the blood bank, recruiting donors, a perfect job for him.

A young lady replaced Suheim as my receptionist in Ras Tanura. Her spoken English was only fair, her written English poor and she had no clinical skills, yet I came to appreciate this sweet girl. Her father had died several years previously so this job was of importance to her and her family, for the extra money would greatly improve their life-style.

Saudi Arabian women, draped from head to toe in black folds of cloth, had seemed forbidding at first. It is easy to be afraid of what you don't see or understand. But I soon found that under those mysterious dark drapes lurked ordinary women, just like me. Women who could easily be coaxed into conversation and laughter, who unfailingly delighted me with their excitement and affection.

I learned a lot about Saudi Arabian women from Zahara. She wore the obligatory black abaya and scarf over her head, but instead of the full-face covering popular in the Eastern Province she wore a veil which covered only her nose and mouth, leaving her eyes exposed. It was a wise choice. She could establish eye contact with a patient, which was important for communication, and yet retain her modesty. I asked her if she minded wearing the mask.

"No," she said. "Because I know myself. I smile too much."

I understood her fear that men would think her smiles were a 'come-on'. I came to know her eyes well—they were large and luminous, full of life and expression. On the few occasions she moved about without the veil—when the unit was empty and she and I were alone—I was surprised and delighted with her smile. She was not 'beautiful,' she had rather heavy features, but her personality shone endearingly. She would have been a gem of a wife and mother and this, as with all Saudi Arabian women, was her dearest wish.

When she first began work with me she spoke of a fiancé. They had been engaged for a long period of time by Saudi Arabian standards, but he was very poor and could not afford the customary dowry or wedding party. So he was saving up. After two years Zahara became impatient.

"I will forgive the dowry and the party," she told him by phone. "I just want to be married."

Their engagement dissolved. Perhaps he did not truly love her or perhaps he felt he would lose face by not giving the traditional gifts. During the years I knew Zahara, there were at least three other suitors who could have made a match with her, but her family vetoed each of them.

"What do Saudi Arabian women think of their husbands marrying a second wife?" I asked her one day.

Her black eyes flashed furiously.

"They don't like it. If they love their husband they don't want to share him with another woman. They spend a lot of money."

A Moslem man must treat all of his wives exactly the same and if his first wife is a big spender he cannot possibly afford another!

Zahara was the youngest in her family. She and I both believed that her family wanted her to remain single to care for her widow mother, and that they would never give permission for another engagement. Her elder sisters and brother were married and had their own families to care for. Zahara's wages helped to run her mother's household and support a lazy brother.

My new receptionist was always anxious to please, and worked hard. She enjoyed the social interaction at work and when the time came for her first annual leave she was reluctant to take it. Once or twice she came into the office just to sit and enjoy the companionship! It was boring at home, she told me, and after she resumed her duties she described to me the highlight of her vacation.

She had persuaded three girlfriends to accompany her on the Aramco bus to the Dhahran compound's beach at Halfmoon Bay. This in itself was impressive, for Saudi Arabian women are not allowed to go anywhere without the permission of their men folk.

The four girls had discarded their abayas and veils and changed into stretch pants and T shirts. They spent the day on the beach where they swam, sang Western songs and spoke only English.

They attracted curious glances from other bathers, but who was to say they were not from Lebanon or some other country where women were not obliged to hide themselves away from the prying eyes of men? I was both amused and saddened by this story. What a pity that the best part of a girl's holiday should be a stolen day at the beach, a pleasure that most of us take for granted.

Zahara asked me one day what she could do at home.

"I get so bored," she said. "I read and I sew, but then I want to do something else and there is nothing. Nothing!"

I suggested a few hobbies but in her situation there really was no answer. She was one of the lucky ones, to have a job and to be able to leave the house and interact with other people. She would dearly have loved to travel and I would have been thrilled to have her come with me on vacation, but her family would never have allowed it.

You could always tell how many wives a man had by watching him in the supermarket. If he picked up two of everything he had two wives. If he picked up four of everything he had four wives. However, in these modern times, it is becoming less common for a man to take more than one wife.

It was considered the height of rudeness to ask a man about his wife, even if it was only to enquire about her health. You could ask about himself or his kids, but never the wife.

An old Saudi Arab patient of mine had only one wife.

"You can't treat four wives the same," he told me. "It's impossible. You can only love one woman. One heart, one woman." What a happy home he must have had!

One of Zahara's would-be suitors had a wife already, but even so she finally decided to accept his proposal. She had to be truly desperate, considering all we had discussed. When her family rejected him also, she was despondent. When I finally left Saudi Arabia she was twenty-two and very definitely on the shelf. Saudi Arabs prefer their wives to be young.

However, Zahara was not to remain single. Some years later I found that she had finally set her sights on a first cousin, a good man who apparently was too shy to make the first advances but who was very happy to become her husband. They now have two children.

Zahara has built a house with an Aramco loan and bought a car. She wields the bulk of the money and most of the power in the relationship but they are a very happy couple.

29 - BIG HILL

MY HEART RACED feebly as wild images ran through my mind. *So this is hallucination.* Mild nausea washed over me. The strange images in my mind slowly subsided, but I could not sleep again, listening instead to the uneasy breathing of my travel companions in the other bunks. In half an hour, at midnight, we would rise for the final onslaught against the summit of the mountain.

To reach the 'roof of Africa'—Kilimanjaro, the highest free standing mountain in the world—had been a dream of mine since childhood. In my fourth year with Aramco, a nurse friend and I decided to make the trip together.

Christine had lived in Kenya for some years and had always wanted to climb the mountain. Rob had climbed it a couple of years previously with a DOG group (Dhahran Outing Group) and I wanted to experience the mountain in the same way that he had experienced it. We contacted a tour company to arrange porters and reserve huts for us on the walk.

The great mountain stands near the border of Tanzania and Kenya, three degrees below the equator, majestic at nineteen thousand, three hundred and forty-two feet above sea level. It is an ancient volcano with three peaks—Mawenzi, Shira and Uhuru (the highest, on Kibo). The snow capped wonder remained unconquered until Hans Meyer made it to the top in 1889.

There is something which draws people to mountaintops, and this one is within the reach of any reasonably fit person. Well-worn paths lure thousands of hopeful tourists here each year, although on average only one in three makes it to the summit. Many factors affect a person's performance along the way.

Acute mountain sickness is the main hazard at these altitudes. The best way to prevent it is to climb slowly, allowing plenty of time for your body to adjust to the altitude, and to eat and drink regularly. Dehydration is a major factor in acute mountain sickness and those who can drink plenty of fluids without retention do better. Hypothermia is also a danger.

Diamox, a medication taken by climbers, is aimed at increasing the flow of fluids through the body. This reduces the risk of cerebral edema, or swelling around the brain. Climbers are urged to go back down the mountain if they experience severe shortness of breath, coughing (especially if the sputum is blood stained), severe headaches, lack of coordination, and hallucinations.

Climbing Kilimanjaro is like traveling from the equator to the arctic in three days. The changes in climate and terrain can produce devastating effects on the human body. Christine and I were determined to make it to the top and took every piece of advice seriously.

It was essential to have medical checkups before getting too far along with travel plans, to exclude medical conditions which might hamper us and to determine which medications and shots we would need. Our respiratory function tests and EKG's revealed no abnormalities, and our blood tests showed good hemoglobin levels.

We decided on mid-January for our trip, as the weather is usually dry and clear then. The Marangu route was our choice of trails, being the most popular and the easiest, with huts to sleep in every night and porters to carry our belongings. The limit for pack weight was thirty pounds. Layers of clothing, warm and wonderfully light, would keep us comfortable all the time we were traveling.

We had started preparations for the climb several months earlier. Christine trained in the gym, while I ran daily. Eventually I could breathe through my nose while running, and then I began running in boots. When January arrived, I could run indefinitely without fatiguing—admittedly only at sea level on flat ground!

Christine and I also paid attention to our diet. If athletes were particular about the food they ate, we reasoned, we could justifiably benefit also and accordingly avoided fats, sugars and high salt foods. Carbohydrates were high on our list; we limited the use of beverages and foods containing caffeine (which promotes dehydration) and drank lots of water.

The flight to Africa left in the evening. Soon after the plane took off from Dhahran airport, it landed in Doha, where we waited for a connecting flight for several hours. The rest of the night slipped away in a blur, sleep interspersed with periods of wakefulness during which both Christine and I craved water. The medication was already at work! Air hostesses stared in astonishment as we drained bottle after bottle of water and asked for more.

Early morning revealed the great continent of Africa beneath us and Christine, who had worked in Kenya before joining Aramco, pointed out the Rift Valley which stretched out its awesome arms below. We circled around the mountains of Kilimanjaro and Kenya before landing late morning. Humid air swirled around us and brightly colored birds twittered excitedly as we walked out of the airport and under the umbrella of a huge flame tree.

Our cheerful driver threw our baggage into the back of a battered white minivan and we piled inside. Eagerly I peered through the window at the countryside flashing by. My main impression was of tropical greenery, and children who ran barefoot around villages; it reminded me of the Pacific islands I'd grown up in.

Mount Meru Game Lodge nestled at the edge of the National Park. Its large gardens attracted many colorful birds and in the grounds wandered zebra, eland, ostriches and a variety of other animals which were supported by the Sanctuary. There were over thirty-three acres of land in the park and signs warned would-be wanderers of the presence of wild animals beyond the park limits. Our room was comfortable and the food good, and we retired early before our big adventure the next day.

In the morning we were driven to Marangu Gate, where the walk started at six thousand, one hundred feet elevation. The terrain was hilly around the base of the mountain and banana and coffee plantations flourished along the curves of the foothills.

After signing in we each rented a ski pole to use as a staff during the climb. Here our guide, Remy, met us. With him were an assistant guide, and four porters to carry our luggage and food for the five days of the trek.

The first section of the trail wound up through gentle rainforest and we needed our rain gear for the light but frequent showers. It was warm and humid under the forest canopy, with a small stream flowing beside the muddy path. Rhododendrons, orchids, violets, and carpets of balsam flourished, and Remy pointed out the *Impatiens Kilimanjari*, a small flower unique to the area. Christine and I checked our pulse rates from time to time when we stopped to rest.

"Can we take your pulse?" Christine asked Remy during one of these sessions.

"No, no!" he replied. "I will carry all the things!"

Trees covered in long vines were home to a large variety of bird life, and hornbills and turacos feasted on the fruit of figs and palms. Birdcalls echoed in the trees, the musty-sweet scent of pink begonia hung on the air and gray-green beards of lichen brushed against us as we walked.

Of all the animals in the jungle, only the monkeys dared to show themselves. Leopards avoided humans. The guides had seen the big cats as high up as twelve thousand five hundred feet, but far away from the camps.

The occasional fallen tree lay across the rainforest path, but the gradient was easy. The most limiting factor was the altitude. *"Pole, pole.* Slowly, slowly," the porters cautioned. From the lowest levels we kept a steady pace, allowing our bodies to gradually adapt to the altitude.

We spent our first night at Mandara camp, nine thousand feet above sea level. The guides dried our damp boots near the fire while we made the short walk up to Maundi Crater, fifteen minutes from Mandara. Each hut slept four but we had one all to ourselves and slept well. The next morning we set off early, our waterbags full.

"I haven't seen you drink anything," I said to Remy. "How much water do you bring with you, for yourself?"

"About half a liter for six of us, two guides and the four porters, going up," he answered. "We drink more coming back."

I wondered if they deprived themselves of liquids to avoid mountain sickness, and what the long-term effects of this would be on their bodies.

Across the rolling heathland, which we entered shortly after leaving Mandara camp, were lovely views of Kibo and Mawenzi peaks. This gave way to moorland with giant lobelias and groundsels. Alpine mist drifted across the landscape. We stopped near a small bush to watch a hyrax busily working its way through the leaves, until it spotted us and disappeared with a flick of its tail.

Conditions on the mountain can change rapidly. The temperature varies from below freezing to very hot, so as well as warm clothing we also needed sunscreen.

The huts at the camp of Horombo were similar to those at Mandara, and snuggled into a hillside dotted with clumps of strange-leafed plants, the giant Senecios. Many people experience headaches, confusion, and shortness of breath on exertion at this altitude. Even some of the young porters had problems on the track between Marangu and Horombo and asked hikers for water.

The porters carried heavy loads—two packs on one head—and many were dressed only in shorts and thongs. The older, more seasoned guides would nonchalantly light up their cigarettes and stride ahead while their charges were gasping for air.

At Horombo, the beauty of the Milky Way was reflected in the myriad of lights in the valleys far below. Sleep was fitful here at twelve thousand five hundred feet and I woke up a couple of times with panic attacks and shortness of breath.

When morning came we noticed a porter hammering at the door of a hut nearby. Eventually he found help and pried the door open. A Japanese lady had died in there during the night. She had felt ill the previous day while walking towards Kibo with her three friends, and had turned back. We saw the rest of her group later that day as they were returning to Horombo and felt sad to think of the news awaiting them.

From Horombo we made our way over high moorlands, the sight of Kibo with its snowy mane beckoning us on. Herds of Eland occasionally roam here, taking advantage of the highest growing vegetation.

We stopped at a small spring marked "Last Water," before continuing across the Saddle, the gently sloping, desolate region between Mawenzie and Kibo, sister peaks of Kilimanjaro. No blade of vegetation grew here on the packed, barren earth. It seemed that nothing could live here, apart from a few small spiders and insects which preferred to crawl rather than to fly. The silence was eerie.

This was a tedious day, broken only by lunch at a huge rock. We dragged ourselves behind this rock for a pit stop, aware that there was no other cover until we reached Kibo hut. My body felt heavy and even the smallest movement seemed to take forever.

At fifteen thousand five hundred and twenty feet above sea level we reached Kibo, the last camp. Its dormitory style rooms each held twelve beds and there was no concession to comfort. There were no ladders to the top bunks and the lower bunks were already occupied by the time we arrived. The seats of the pit toilets outside were spattered with frozen vomit, from those already suffering from the altitude.

It was all we could do to haul ourselves up to our bunks and change our clothes for the night. *What a waste of space and weight bringing books to read.* I forced myself to write a little in my diary before collapsing from exhaustion. Sleep would not come and I checked my watch frequently until our wake-up call at eleven thirty pm.

The plan was to leave camp at midnight. First we gathered in the dining area to eat breakfast. After a few mouthfuls, sour orange and stale toast surged upward in my throat and I struggled out of my seat, stumbled outside and threw up. Soon our guides led us off into the blackness. It was actually a relief to be upright and to be able to breathe a little easier. Now we wore all our warmest layers of clothing. It was very cold and some of the other travelers' water bottles froze.

According to the guidebooks, one of the reasons for leaving at this time is that the scree up the slopes toward the crater rim is frozen and easier to walk on at this time. Another reason is that the sight of the steep ascent above you is not so daunting in the dark!

Up the slope we trudged, small switchbacks behind the guide easier than a direct ascent. You can do anything for an hour. And then another. *Breathe and step...breathe and step...*I focused numbly on the boots in front of mine, focused on my feelings. You live on the edge in this moon-walk, only a breath away from mountain sickness.

Falling stars were common and the Southern Cross sparkled above, a reminder that we were in the Southern Hemisphere. At Hans Meyer's Cave, the halfway point, we sat down to rest. Christine lay down but was quickly roused by the guide, who was afraid she might drift into a coma.

We staggered off again into the night. *Breathe and step...breathe and step...*Then sunrise began to transform the mountain; the growing sunlight cast a ruddy glow over the world and we saw that the scree was giving way to rocky outcrops. The rising sun appeared far below on the horizon, and rapidly ascended to reveal an overwhelming panorama.

"Makes the past six hours seem like just a bad dream, doesn't it," I whispered. My voice sounded tinny to my own ears.

"No," Christine croaked. I looked at her in the pale yellow light. She looked ill and I felt a pang of alarm.

"Are you OK?" I asked.

"I can hardly breathe and there are spots in front of my eyes," she said miserably. She *had* to make it; we couldn't come this far without at least getting to the rim of the crater.

"Rest a minute or two and just concentrate on your breathing," I said. "We can take our time. Look! There's Gilman's Point up there, see where those people are standing?"

Just then a man staggered past us on the way down, his face pallid. He was wrapped in a space blanket and was supported by a thin, worried-looking guide.

"Do I look like that?" Christine asked anxiously.

"No," I said. Her skin was blanched and her eyes were dull, but there was expression in her face.

Little by little we inched upward. Gilman's Point, at eighteen thousand, six hundred and forty feet, is for many the end of the journey. Even for those who can go no further, this point is a momentous achievement and a certificate is issued. Here the guides sing a special song—the song of Kilimanjaro.

I took Christine's photo in front of the Gilman sign, then hugged her and watched sadly as she began the long descent, accompanied by Remy's assistant. From the very beginning we had made a pact that if one of us had to give up the other would continue, but I couldn't help feeling guilty all the same.

Remy and I turned to go on. It was another seven hundred and twelve vertical feet up Kibo's breast to Uhuru, the highest point on the mountain. There was a reverent feeling in the air. Someone else must have thought so too, for etched in elegant script on a rock were the words, *'All the earth worships Thee; they sing praises to Thy name. Psalm 66/3'*.

Hot sulphurous gases floated up from the ash pit in the cone at the center of the crater. The volcano was only sleeping. Here the snow was deeper and the pathway wiggled treacherously along the crater's edge.

Then suddenly we arrived, at nineteen thousand three hundred and forty two feet above sea level. The peak with its glacial band glowed greenly in the sunlight; Mawenzi and the valleys below were part of an awesome panorama. For several minutes I wandered in a daze before joining the short line of successful climbers waiting to write their names in the book of achievers. It was hard to unwind my cold fingers from the pen after the effort.

"We have to go, quickly! You must not stay here long." Remy allowed me only a few minutes at the summit. It was dangerous to stay up here for too long.

After descending carefully to Gilman's Point, we bounded down the scree like puppies on a sand dune, back toward Horombo where Christine was waiting. The heaviness and malaise miraculously disappeared as we lost altitude and only then did the exhilaration begin—we had reached the roof of Africa!

Every memorable event in my life has prompted me to write poetry, and I was compelled to write this of Kilimanjaro:

> Queen of peaks, you beckon me, your icy crown above the sky.
>
> All silent broods your dormant breast; your presence Majesty.
>
> How elegant your tresses green, where bounty of the forest grows.
>
> Now dare I tread your paths unseen, your heart to know.
>
> Capricious mistress! Who can bear to tell of those whose breath—whose very life—you snatched, who tried to gain your summit fair?
>
> What secrets guard you on the trail? Uhuru's ground I must acquaint.
>
> My spirit wanes, my heart grows faint, for life is frail.
>
> Through the swirling mists I climb to shining green of glacier's shelf.
>
> Here I must revelation find—my friend, my foe, my self.
>
> Desperate clings my soul to life, the monarch knows.
>
> Then sunrise glows on Kibo's brow and we who toiled through darkest night may greet the dawn,
>
> Triumphant now.

Back in Ras Tanura, work was anticlimactic. For months we'd planned and trained and now it was all over. To add to the gloom, my fortieth birthday arrived the week we returned to Ras Tanura. When you are ten years old, the world is before you and twenty seems impossibly ancient. At twenty, you're busy trying to find a niche to fit into. At thirty you're comfortable in your chosen career and hopefully in your social life. At forty, you realize you are on the downhill run. You find yourself thinking back on things as much as thinking forward and start to wonder if you missed something along the way.

"Happy birthday to you!" A voice on the phone sang, just after I got up on the morning of my birthday.

"Tanya!" I exclaimed. "Thanks very much. You know it's my fortieth. I'm trying to forget it."

"Ha! Ha!" she laughed. "We're taking you out to dinner tonight, around six o'clock. You'd better be ready!"

Later Christine called to say that we girls would meet at her place for drinks and nibbles and then Rob would take us all to Rahima for a meal. Rob's house was in darkness when we arrived, but as we rang the doorbell and pushed open the front door every light in the house went on and twenty people yelled, "*Surprise!*"

When you are depressed about turning forty, a surprise party is a very nice thing. The shock of adrenaline carries you over the threshold into a new decade and reminds you of the many friends you have who are already there and are still enjoying life.

Penny Hamilton wore a T shirt that said, "It is better to be over the hill than under it," and Gerry and Jackie gave me a fake fur hat with built-in ear muffs. There were many other useless and garish gifts which made me laugh until the tears ran and I discovered that while I was off climbing the highest free-standing mountain in the world, friends were cooking up my favorite foods for this night.

They had also ordered a special cake in the shape of Kilimanjaro, decorated with climbers, skiers and reminders of other activities I enjoyed. Truly, I was fortunate to have so many wonderful people around me.

30 - BACK IN THE SAND PIT

"WHAT ARE YOU doing?"

I spun around, shocked. The Saudi Arabian policeman, in full uniform, had arrived unnoticed. I stared at my feet, knowing full well that what we were doing was illegal.

The others in our group realized, one by one, that we had a visitor and the chatter petered out, replaced by a guilty silence.

"We're just looking for those," someone said eventually, pointing to the rocky piles by the back of the vehicle.

Occasionally expatriates came to this patch of the desert to dig for sand roses. These beautiful crystals are the color of the sand they grow in, and develop two to four feet below the surface in moist areas where there is a high concentration of calcium carbonate. The crystals grow singly or in clusters, and can be so large and heavy that they are difficult to retrieve without damage. Most look like roses, hence the name.

The policeman stared in astonishment.

"What is this?" he asked excitedly. "I have never seen anything like this before!"

We explained how the crystals grew; they were soft at first but became as hard as rock on maturing.

"Can I help you dig?" asked the policeman. "I would like to find some too."

"Of course!"

We were delighted to show him how to dig for the crystals, scooping and brushing away the sand until they could be lifted out undamaged.

Saudi Arabian officials later withdrew their taboo on collecting sand roses, as it was discovered that they grew much faster than previously thought. There was no great loss to the country if a few expatriates dug for them once in a while.

My assistant, Suheim, was intrigued by our adventures in the desert.

"My family owns a very old village near Buraydah," he said. "Nobody lives there now and I have never been there myself. When King Abdul Aziz came through that area long ago he stayed there. If you are ever up that way, can you look for it?"

One weekend we headed northwest, specifically to find Suheim's village. In Buraydah, we stopped to ask someone if he knew anything about the old village. While Rob was talking, another man came along. He was obviously a mutawa, by his short thowb and long, bushy beard.

"Salaam," said Rob, offering his hand through the window.

The old man looked at us long and hard, keeping his own hand behind his back.

"*Mafi Moslem, mafi salaam,* No welcome for a non-Moslem," he said at last.

Rob was speechless; it was the only time in Arabia that he had experienced a rebuff like this.

Nobody seemed to know anything about Suheim's old village. We drove all day, criss-crossing the region, searching for the elusive ruins. Towards sunset we were lucky enough to find someone who remembered it and could give directions—it turned out to be close to where we had begun our search!

Stepping back into the past, we imagined the village as it must have been and how the people would have thrilled at the visit of King Abdul Aziz. It was worth our time to see Suheim's face aglow with pleasure when we told him of our discovery and handed him the photos we had taken.

When Rob mentioned the incident with the unfriendly mutawa, Suheim was aghast. This man was not a good Moslem, he said; those who practice Islam should *always* return a greeting.

I was nervous at check points, especially around Buraydah which was a strict fundamentalist area. Even in convoy it could be considered an offense for an unmarried couple to travel unchaperoned in a vehicle together.

At one checkpoint, Rob showed his *iqama* at the request of the attendant official. A married man always had his wife's picture on his *iqama*. Here was a problem—Rob's *iqama* contained no hint of a wife.

So who was I? I produced my own *iqama* and held my breath for the reaction. The officer paused a moment.

"Sister, right?" he said in Arabic, waving us on with a grin.

One Eid, Rob invited both Tanya and me on a camping trip. This time the three of us went in one vehicle; the roads were good and well-traveled in the area and we felt no need of company.

Again we had to pass through Buraydah and we girls began to sweat as Rob pulled to a halt at the checkpoint. The officer in charge beckoned for Rob's *iqama*. Then mine. Then Tanya's. He looked at each of the documents, perplexed. *All different names?*

Rob shrugged.

"Under Islamic law I am allowed four wives," he answered in Arabic, "I only have two!"

The officer doubled up, laughing. He pumped Rob's hand vigorously. His assistant, also laughing, stuck his hand in the window to shake hands too. A quiet demeanor, a bit of humor and a good command of Arabic combined to set officials at ease. They really did not want trouble if it could be avoided.

These were unforgettable days in the desert. In the midst of total isolation we could happen onto an ancient Turkish fort or abandoned village which was gradually giving way to the relentless ravages of the desert.

Sometimes there were treasures worth salvaging—hand-painted doors and windows, old brass pots, cauldrons and other hardware, awaiting inevitable burial in the drifting sand. Romans had also passed this way and occasionally a bronze coin or

Roman arrowhead would be sighted. In the desert areas close to the gulf it is possible to stumble upon ruins left over from the slave trade—old custom houses, pottery shards and ancient beads, evidence of habitation long ceased.

Nothing was fenced. The Bedou roamed free and so did we, stopping at will to rest, take photographs or play on sand dunes. There was no greater freedom in the world. It was no wonder that the nomads refused all attempts to settle them in fixed housing.

The King himself once ordered the construction of massive blocks of apartments for the people of the desert. But the buildings were never occupied; the Bedou preferred their desert haunts to being cooped up in a housing development. I couldn't blame them.

Other secrets of the windswept plains included flint arrowheads. To hold a piece of finely chiseled stone, last held by another hand thousands of years previously, filled me with a sense of awe. I hunted for arrowheads as avidly as any other expatriate, training my eye until I could spot a promising shape at the windward edge of a dune. The beautiful stone tools were fashioned by flaking, and displayed excellent craftsmanship—I could only imagine the hands that had fashioned them and the game they attempted to kill—to hold history in your hand is a wonderful feeling.

I developed another method of hunting for arrowheads. Placing my hands flat on the hard ground immediately in front of a dune, I pressed them down under the loose sand of the slip face. Arrowheads were readily identifiable and I found most of my collection that way. Other expats may have plucked the visible areas clean but under the dunes was virgin territory laden with treasures.

Fossils also abounded. Our favorite haunts included the Mastodon Bones where a herd of ancient animals had been suddenly entombed, their huge tusks and bones visible in crumbling rock faces and overhangs. There was also Shark Tooth Wadi, a valley with shells, and shark teeth of many sizes and shapes.

One day Tanya showed me a package which she had brought back from Thailand.

"Look—Saudi diamonds!" she said, her eyes shining. "Aren't they gorgeous? I picked the stones up from the ground on a camping trip and had them cut when I went to Bangkok."

The glittering cut stones were magnificent.

"Where did you find them?" I asked eagerly.

"*Qasumah*," she replied. "They are everywhere—just off the road. You can spot them easily, all over the surface of the ground."

Soon I had my own collection of Saudi or *Qasumah* diamonds, which are not real diamonds at all but very hard quartz. In Thailand, for two or three dollars apiece, these stones can be transformed into lovely gems. After they have been cut and heat-treated, only a jeweler with an eye-piece can distinguish them from the real thing and many girls have had them made into jewelry.

One Eid holiday I went again with Rob, Brian and Dani to the caves in *Ma'aqala*. As well as our geological discoveries we found three young owlets, hidden in rocky overhangs at the top of a high *jebel* or hill. The fluffy chicks gazed at us with wide golden eyes, hissing softly as their parents called anxiously from across the valley.

On our last morning at camp I woke up to the sounds of someone lighting the fire and filling the tea kettle. The air in my tent was warming up in the rays of the morning sun, and I savored the last moments of rest for soon it would be too hot to remain inside.

Suddenly a gunshot broke the silence. Then another. What on earth was going on? A few moments later a cheery voice called out. I unzipped the fly of my tent an inch and pressed one eye to the opening. A short, bearded Saudi Arab in a dirty white *thowb* extended his right hand to shake Rob's. From his other hand dangled a dead pigeon. Several camels jostled behind him.

"We have been shooting pigeons," he announced. "We have twenty."

"Twenty!" said Rob, impressed. "That's a lot of pigeons."

"Yes," continued the Arab. "We eat a lot of them. How do you like my camels?"

"Very nice," said Rob. "Are they good camels?"

"Ah yes!" said the Arab. "Camels are wonderful animals. If you treat them well, they will treat you well also."

I had heard camels bray, but I had never seen one spit or behave aggressively.

"Would you like to come and join us for *kabsa* today?" asked our visitor.

Of course we would, thank you very much, and shortly before lunchtime found our way to the large white villa owned by our new friend. He ushered us into the cool *majlis*, the meeting room, where we sank gratefully onto a red carpeted floor and leaned back onto heavy cushions.

Our congenial host beckoned his sons to serve us coffee in small, thimble-shaped cups, then heavily sugared tea and fresh dates. I was beginning to like fresh dates. They were infinitely better than dried dates, especially when only half ripened and still a little crunchy at one end.

Dani and I sat slightly apart from the men and whispered softly together in English while the men spoke in Arabic of their camels and their children, and of how many birds they had shot that morning. In turn, Rob and Brian explained why we were camping that weekend and described the caves we had come to explore. The Arabs were fascinated. They only valued caves for the water they may contain, or as dumping grounds for dead sheep and old engine oil.

Suddenly one of the young men motioned to Dani and me.

"Come, I will take you to the ladies," he said.

At the rear of the house was another building where ten or fifteen women waited, along with several children of varying ages. Their *majlis* was bare, apart from the carpeted floor. They were all as excited as a kindergarten class, and had obviously been expecting us.

They stroked our hair and arms, laughing and chattering amongst themselves. Then they bombarded us with questions. Before long my brain was throbbing with the effort of thinking in Arabic and translating for Dani, who had less knowledge of the language than I.

We were both very hungry when the meal arrived. The men would have eaten first as was the custom, and afterward the meal would have been re-shaped and added to for the rest of us.

The platter of seasoned rice smelled wonderful but I tried not to look at the cluster of scrawny, dark-fleshed birds in the centre of the plate. Their legs and heads were intact; scorched eyeballs stared accusingly at us. I concentrated mainly on the rice which was moist and delicious with the *kabsa* spices.

From time to time the chief hostess would wrench a choice morsel of meat from a fragile skeleton and toss it across to the space in front of me or Dani. I knew that this was a courtesy I could not refuse, and tried to be gracious about the gifts as they arrived. The meat tasted gamey but was quite palatable.

After the meal we were again plied with questions, and entered into a spirited discussion of marriage, children, and our countries of origin. It was easy to warm to these people, with their child-like curiosity about the world beyond their confines and their eagerness to accept us as friends.

As the afternoon was ageing I suggested it may be time to move on.

"No!" they insisted. "Your husbands are sleeping now; wait until they wake up!"

With difficulty we tore ourselves away and returned to the main *majlis*, where the men were actually waiting, and wondering what had happened to us!

Out in the desert, near the port city of *Jubail*, was a high wire fence erected by the Department of Saudi Antiquities. The fence enclosed the remains of ancient buildings, which had been discovered in the mid 1980's by someone trying to dig his vehicle out of the sand. The ruins are those of a church and its surrounds, and the Department of Antiquities will not issue permits to visit because they say it is "being excavated."

Independent reports reveal that this church is probably the oldest in the world and was most likely built under a Nestorian bishopric which existed in the area in the fourth century. Around the walls of the old building were distinct niches the shape of crosses, and these were originally filled with stone crosses which have since gone missing.

On my first visit to the church I was able to scramble under the fence and walk around amongst the ruins. By my second visit, several years later, someone had tried their best to obliterate the outline of the crosses by chipping at them with a sharp instrument. The Department of Antiquities had replaced the old fence with a sturdy new one which was impossible to breach, but there had been no attempts at further excavation. Now that the building is exposed to the atmosphere it will probably deteriorate.

The desert itself was the greatest treasure of all. Sometimes my heart would ache with the peace and sense of timelessness I found there. And the friends we made amongst the Bedou made our experiences very precious indeed.

31 - GATED!

ONE THURSDAY I was visiting Rob when he got a phone call from the computer store in Rahima, telling him that his repaired computer was ready. The Filipinos from the store had brought it to the gate.

They were, however, unable to enter as they didn't have sufficient identification to satisfy the security guards at the gate. Could Rob please come and pick it up from them outside the gate?

But Rob had only just driven off when he walked back into the house.

"What? Back so soon?" I asked.

"You're going to have to take me," he said. "My car died just around the corner."

Chad and Naomi were on leave and as I was house-sitting for them I had the use of Naomi's car. Rob asked me to drive.

"We'll have to switch seats here," I said, as we neared the compound gate. "They won't let me drive through the gate you know."

"That's OK," said Rob, "Keep driving."

"They'll stop us!" I protested.

Sure enough, as we drew alongside the gate, the security guard motioned to me to get out of the car. His English was almost non-existent but his intention was clear. We changed seats and Rob drove out of the gate and around the corner to the car park.

This gate was different from the other entrances to camp. The clinics were on the other side of this gate and so the road for some distance to the perimeter fence was still on Aramco property. However the rules were the same—women were not to drive outside the gates.

Rob paid the Filipinos and lifted the computer into the back seat. Then he turned to me.

"You drive back into camp."

"I can't do that! The guard won't like that at all."

"They didn't say you couldn't drive *into* the compound," he said impishly, "They only said you couldn't drive *out!*"

Reluctantly I climbed into the driver's seat and, as I expected, was stopped at the gate. The security supervisor had arrived and reprimanded me sternly. His English was good.

"You must not drive outside this gate," he said. "Someone might see you and it would not be a good thing for them to see a lady driving outside this gate."

I nodded humbly and we were allowed to leave.

"What could I have done if I had been the one collecting the computer?" I wondered, on the way back to Rob's house. "If I had no male contact to help me drive through the gate, I'd be out of luck. I couldn't walk with that computer through the gate to the car! You know, there really should be some kind of a neutral zone adjoining Aramco property, where single women can conduct business like this."

I let it slide for a couple of weeks, but finally got around to writing a letter to Security to make this proposition. A couple of days later at work I had a phone call. It was Abdullah, the Saudi Arab in charge of Government Affairs. He had been a patient of mine and I was currently treating his mother.

"Hey, Abdullah!" I said. "What can I do for you?"

"Well, Judy," he said, "I've called because I need you to come to a meeting here in my office."

"Oh really," I said. "What about?"

"I'll tell you when you arrive."

"Oh. Well...how about...Wednesday. I can clear some time on my schedule by then."

"That's too late," he said. "I was thinking of this afternoon at twelve thirty."

"Hmmm. I guess I can reschedule a few patients. How long will the meeting be?"

"About an hour, I think. There will be officers from Personnel and Security as well as myself."

"That sounds serious!" I said with a lurch of apprehension.

"It is," he replied.

I had always been careful to comply with regulations since entering this country. What had I done wrong?

Quickly I re-arranged my schedule, and got away from the clinic in plenty of time. When I arrived at Abdullah's office I was glad to see May, his secretary. May and I had been on a ski holiday with an Aramco group and knew each other well.

"Do you know why this meeting has been called?" I asked her.

"Ohhh! I could lose my job if I tell you," she whispered looking furtively around, "but—it's because you drove through the gate."

I chuckled. "Is that all! Thanks for warning me!"

Soon Abdullah arrived and ushered me into his office. I was pleased to see that the Personnel officer was Chuck, a friendly American who was well liked by Saudi Arabs and expats alike. There was also a security officer, who didn't appear to understand much English. In Arabic fashion, we exchanged pleasantries for several minutes before getting down to business.

Abdullah set the ball rolling.

"Three weeks ago a car stopped at the gate near the clinic. A young lady was driving and there was a man in the passenger seat. The guard on duty made them change seats so the man could drive out of the gate. A little while later the car came back in again, and the young lady was at the wheel! This time the supervisor was present and he told her she should not be doing this. He took the details of the car but he did not ask her for her ID.

"When he reported this incident we realized that it was Naomi Anderson's car, but Naomi was of course on vacation, so who could be driving her car? For three weeks we have been trying to find out who was driving Naomi's car!"

"Ahhh!" I exclaimed. "And then you got my letter."

"Then we got your letter," said Abdullah. "You solved the mystery for us."

"Well I'm so glad I was able to help," I said. "And by the way, why *is* there a problem with women driving through that gate—why can't there be a neutral zone in that car park so that single females can conduct business? What if a girl had to pick up a computer and had no man to drive her?"

"The security officer would be able to drive her car around," said Abdullah.

"But what if the security officer doesn't speak English?" I asked. "And besides, isn't it still Aramco property on the other side of the gate, between the gate and the clinic?"

"Yes, but you can't drive out there. There's nothing to stop you—you might just keep on driving, out to the highway."

"Oh I wouldn't want to do that," I said. "Too much traffic on that road. I would just want to get to that car park. Anyway I always thought females were allowed to drive on Aramco property."

"You know, the area on both sides of the pipeline all around Arabia is Aramco property. The line between RT and Dhahran is Aramco property."

"Ohhhh!" I exclaimed. "That means I could..."

"No Judy!" said Abdullah, his lips twitching. "That does *not* mean you can drive along the pipeline to Dhahran from here!"

I grinned. Chuck was choking.

I fell back on the explanation which all Saudi Arabs understand—and which, in fact was the truth.

"Actually, I didn't want to drive through the gate. The man who was with me *told* me to drive back through the gate. He made me do it. What else could I do?" I raised my arms in a gesture of helplessness.

Abdullah nodded.

"OK. But you should not ever drive through the gates again."

"I won't," I said. "But what *does* a single woman do if she needs to conduct business on the other side of the gate, and doesn't have a man to drive her?"

"The security guard could drive you," Abdullah repeated, "and if he could not, then he would call someone to do the job."

There was no answer as to what could be done if the security guard on duty could not speak English.

"I guess that is all then," said Abdullah. "Thank you for coming and I'll see you again sometime. By the way, my mother is coming to see you this afternoon. Look after her please!"

"I will," I promised as I headed out the door.

May had been listening through the wall and raised her fingers in a victory sign. A wide smile filled her face.

The next morning Abdullah called again.

"After you left, Judy, we discussed your case, and we decided that it was not your fault that you drove through the gate. It was the fault of the man who made you do it." There was a long pause.

"Now, Judy, we want to know who that man was who made you drive through the gate."

"Oh Abdullah," I said, "I can't tell you that! Let's just leave it, shall we?"

"Judy," he said, "I'll come to your house at six o'clock and pull out your fingernails!" There was a chuckle in his voice.

"No Abdullah," I said. "I'm not going to tell you, so that's that! Just finish the report and forget about it. Please."

"OK," he said.

What has always puzzled me is this—why could Personnel not simply have looked up the housing papers, which had been signed by both Naomi and me, to find out the identity of the one driving her car that day?

32 - RAVENS, RATS AND SAUDI CATS

RAVENS BRED PROFUSELY on the camps, having an excellent supply of water and no natural predators. Aramco compounds were oases, with gardens and lawns watered by sprinklers on timers and tended by fleets of Indian and Pakistani gardeners—perfect havens for birds.

The greenery ended abruptly at the boundary walls, and from there on white sand and scrub stretched on as far as the eye could see. The ravens were raucous birds, and very aggressive during the nesting season. One almost knocked me off my bike once, as I rode home from work.

Several Texans offered to shoot them, if someone would provide the rifles! At one point there was a rumor that Community Services had contemplated erecting a large net across Surf Avenue to "catch" the birds.

Pest Control tried poisoning the ravens from time to time by placing bait for them in fenced off areas. This cut the numbers back but there was a risk that bait dropped mid-flight might be eaten by pets on camp. At least two dogs I knew had succumbed to this fate. The ravens ruled the air but there was also the occasional parrot, which had escaped from custody and found a pleasant home in the treetops.

Migratory birds on their way between the Northern and Southern hemispheres often visited Aramco camps, green and lush in comparison with their desert surroundings. These birds also provided opportunities for bird watchers. I was once delighted by a pair of long-tailed parrots, which settled for a short while in a tree outside my house.

Often when tripping around the desert one would see a solitary bird in these harsh dry areas—a friend once observed an eagle nest on top of an eight-foot pole. There was nothing higher for him to build on. I guess he knew the meaning of loneliness.

There was other wildlife around, and I once suspected that mice were at work in my apartment. One morning very early, loud gnawing sounds from the ground floor woke me up from a sound sleep. If it was a mouse it was a mighty big one. The next evening I opened my front door to hear rustling in the pantry. Quietly I crept along the passageway until I found the light switch and the pantry door.

One...two...three...now! I switched the light on and flung the pantry door open at the same instant. A huge rat hurtled through the air just inches from my nose, hit the floor running and shot under the oven before my scream had died away.

The next day Pest Control laid two rat traps, baited with peanut butter, in the house. "We will catch it," they assured me and sure enough, before the day was out it was dead. It measured twenty-one inches from the tip of its nose to the tip of its tail, a fine looking animal. I almost felt sorry for my part in its murder.

Wild cats roamed the camp at night. Saudi cats, we called them. These feral animals survived by eating vermin and stealing scraps. They were vicious and strong but they didn't tackle rats. Considering the size of the rat in my apartment I could understand their reservations. From time to time expats made pets of these cats, but there was always a wild streak in the creatures and they could never be completely tamed.

One day a Saudi tabby cat gave birth to two kittens somewhere behind a huge Bougainvillea bush in Rob's backyard. When I first saw them they were a few weeks old. They were obviously sired by a Siamese tomcat, having cream fur with chocolate points. One kitten disappeared but the other grew, nurtured by its fearsome mother.

The kitten became bolder and bolder, although the mother remained wild. She would hiss and spit and come close enough to swat the milk container out of Rob's hand as he poured milk into a bowl for her.

The day came when the mother cat left on a mission with another tomcat, leaving the kitten behind. "Hobie Cat," became his name, as sailing the small catamaran had become an important weekend pastime for us by now.

Hobie was a serious kitten. He never played like other kittens but became very devoted to me and would sit on my lap, gazing up with absolute trust in his blue eyes. Rob teased him mercilessly, so the cat always kept a wary eye on Rob when he was in the same room. At any sign of a visitor he was away, and few others ever saw him.

Cats also lived in the towns, or rather, *existed,* for they were miserable specimens, flea-bitten and starving. Many expats harbored sympathy for the cats. A vet in Al Khobar neutered cats for free and an organization called PAWS developed, which cared for many sick, abandoned and injured animals.

As for wild creatures, there were fox in the desert, along with lizards, falcons, and snakes. Often Rob and I would spend hours observing and deciphering the tracks on the dunes—a notorious and deadly sidewinder, an industrious dung beetle, a shy fox.

If you left your camping supplies out in the night there would be evidence of tiny *jacoba* mice having found the bounty. The *dhub,* a large lizard, sunned itself not far from its burrow, enjoying even the hottest days. Saudi Arabs swore that each part of the creature tasted like a different type of meat. And then there was the desert Saluki, a dog much like our greyhounds—slender, pretty and fast as a whip.

At one time oryx roamed the plains but these became extinct many years before I arrived in Saudi Arabia. During the 1990's a herd of oryx was reintroduced to the southern desert and was reportedly doing well, although those in the know kept the whereabouts of the animals secret for fear they would be hunted.

Scorpions would occasionally burrow under a camper's groundsheet. They were generally placid creatures and would not become irritable unless disturbed, generally happy to trundle around on their own business.

The story was told of an employee who had been living in temporary accommodation and woke up one morning with an eye swollen shut. He suspected that something had bitten him in the night. A few days later after the swelling had gone down, he realized that a piece of skin had gone from under his eye. That afternoon he dropped a pack of cigarettes near the bed and as he stooped to pick it up something rushed out to attack his hand.

He chased the creature and beat it to death, but salvaged the body to show to someone who could identify it. It was a camel spider. These grotesque creatures leap up onto the bodies of camels and other mammals, inject a little local anesthetic and proceed to suck blood and eat small sections of the soft tissues of their host. After these revelations I felt happier using a tent, rather than a cot, in the open air of the desert.

I had the opportunity to see a camel spider in a dry aquarium on camp. The folks at the house showed me the spider, which was destined to be entombed in a glass paperweight. It was the ugliest thing I had ever seen. The body was round and fleshy, perhaps an inch and a half in diameter, the thorax was a third of the size and the head a little smaller still. It had large hairy legs, and a beak with fangs. The whole creature was the size of my palm. As I watched in fascination, someone threw a small fish into the aquarium. The spider threw itself at the fish, clamped its fangs around it and sucked it dry.

My most exciting animal experience in Saudi Arabia occurred during a Scout excursion in the mountains of the *Asir*. One evening as I rested quietly by the fire watching the flames, a movement on the other side of the fire caught my attention. And then I saw it—a Caracal Lynx. I froze, elation and panic vying for priority. For a long moment the large cat stood by the bushes, its gaze locked onto mine. Then it vanished without a sound.

33 - ON THE MAT

PAT HAD GONE on repat and things were crazy in the Physical Therapy unit. Referrals were flooding in like autumn leaves in a stiff breeze. It was all I could do to keep the place running smoothly and Zahara called me into the office more and more frequently to pacify angry patients who could not be seen for several weeks.

Then I was sent a referral for a man who'd had a stroke three years previously. The patient's relatives were unyielding. They wanted an appointment and they wanted it *now*. Zahara and I tried every tactic we knew to persuade them to wait. I called the Filipina doctor who had seen the old man in Emergency.

"Do you think this patient is an urgent case?"

"No," she said. "He had his stroke three years ago, but the family wants him to have treatment so I thought maybe you could evaluate him and see what you could do. He has been in hospital recently but there hasn't really been any change in his condition."

"So is it OK if I give him an appointment in three weeks' time? I have a lot of other acute patients and if he's chronic..."

"Sure," she said. "Three weeks would be fine."

"Three weeks it is," I said to Zahara. "Now I have to get back to work."

She was unable to pacify the patient's relatives and sent them to Fahad in Medical Liaison. Fahad was a wonderful man, well versed in patient psychology and able to calm the most agitated person.

Half an hour later I was called to the phone. It was Dr Aman, the emergency physician.

"I have a patient here who came to see you this afternoon," he said. "He had a stroke and he needs an early appointment with you. His relatives are very concerned about him."

"I spoke with Dr Arena and she says it is not urgent," I said.

"But he will have spasticity if you leave him for three weeks. Can't you see him now?"

"I understand that he had his stroke three years ago," I said, "and I don't believe he is an acute case."

"But he has been in hospital recently. You should see him right now."

I drew a deep breath. Three patients were now waiting in cubicles, at least two more in the waiting area and my blood pressure was rising.

"I'm sorry but I can't spare any more time right now," I said. "I have made an appointment for him. He is also on my priority waiting list. I feel the same as you do—I would like to see every patient as soon as they come in but it's just not possible! I hate sending patients away like this too. Please call my supervisor in Dhahran if you want to discuss this further. Here's her phone number—."

I had a forlorn hope that the increasing numbers of calls to Mary would prompt her to send help sooner rather than later—although of course I knew she was already doing the best she could with limited staff numbers.

I ended up seeing the old patient earlier than the three weeks promised. As I expected, he was not an acute case. The family was pushy, even with the old man, hustling him, urging him and jostling him until he fumbled and almost lost his balance.

He was slow and uncertain but could move around with a walking aid when he was encouraged and given time, so I gave him home exercises and a walking frame and told the family I would see him again after a week of exercise. His condition would not change much.

A few weeks later Dr Desa, the current Chief Physician of the clinics, called me.

"I would like you to come to a meeting in my office next Tuesday afternoon. We need to discuss how we can improve patient relations in Physical Therapy."

"Sure," I answered, taking a look at the schedule. "I can be there."

My heart thumped painfully. I was getting palpitations now, every time my schedule was forced.

I mentioned the planned meeting in a memo to Mary and she called me back.

"Have you discussed this meeting with your medical liaison officer?"

"That's Dr Burg, the American doctor, but he's just gone on vacation this week," I answered. "I think one of the others is standing in for him."

"In that case I should come up for the meeting."

"Is that necessary? I mean, you're very busy too and I don't think it's a big deal. I would probably be OK on my own."

"Well I am coming anyway." Mary sighed. "You might need some support."

Tuesday arrived and Mary came in on the bus as I was sending the last patient out for the morning. We went up to the Surf House for lunch.

"You should bring a pen and paper, and plan to take minutes," she told me.

"Don't you think they will take the minutes?" I asked, surprised.

"I don't think so," she said.

Either she knew something I didn't or she was being paranoid. I shrugged.

"OK, I'll take writing materials."

We arrived at the administration office to find that, as well as Dr Desa, others were present at this meeting—Dr Ibn Aljam as the stand-in Physician Liaison officer, Dr Aman from Emergency, Fahd from Medical Liaison, and Faisal the Clinic Administrator.

Hmmm. Looks like males against the females, I thought. I'll bet they waited for Dr Burg to go on leave before they called this meeting.

If they were surprised that Mary had come too, they hid it well. I took out my pen and paper as we began, for it seemed that Mary was correct—nobody else was going to take the minutes of this meeting.

It all started very cordially. Dr Desa said that past issues should not be dwelt on, but that the future should be looked to in establishing satisfactory methods of dealing with patient complaints before they got out of hand. He said that patient relations were very important, and all our efforts should be directed towards improving quality of patient care, with the emphasis on working as a team. Nobody could argue with that.

Then he said that he would like the Liaison Physician to be involved in prioritizing the P.T. schedule so that problems could be resolved in Ras Tanura and not taken to Dhahran.

Mary responded by handing Dr Desa a copy of an item from the Aramco operating manual.

"This says that the role of the Liaison Physician does not include giving assistance in managing therapists' schedules," she said. "And there is also this one, which gives directives for solving patient complaints—the problem goes to the Rehabilitation Supervisor if it is unable to be resolved locally by the Physical Therapist, the referring Physican, and Medical Liaison."

Dr Desa had no answer. I sensed that he was angry and things started to heat up. One by one, the men had their say but Mary was prepared for battle and had a courteous answer ready for every comment.

"I have had a lot of problems with Judy," Dr Ibn Aljam said suddenly.

It was untrue and so unfair. Mary kicked me under the table and later said she was trying to prevent me retaliating. But I was speechless.

"Well, I also was very unhappy with the bad words I heard on the telephone, when I was trying to get an appointment for the old man," said Dr Aman.

Mary jumped on it.

"What exactly were those bad words?" she demanded. "This sounds like an attitude problem that should be dealt with."

Dr Aman stammered an inadequate response, and I quietly repeated my side of the conversation as best I could remember it.

"That doesn't sound like bad words to me," Mary countered.

"Well there were disgusting passages in the memos she sent me," Dr Desa added.

I was stunned. It was unbelievable, these lies. What on earth was motivating these people? Why did they have such hatred for me? All I had done was to try to cope with an impossible workload.

"Please be specific," Mary said. "I would like to know just what you found disgusting."

A copy of the memo was produced, and Mary shook her head.

"I find nothing disgusting in this."

My head was spinning; my hand shaking so badly that the notes were almost illegible by the time Dr Desa adjourned the meeting. He was coming off poorly and obviously thought it wise to quit while he still had a shred of dignity.

My heart was pounding an irregular tattoo as we walked away from the meeting.

"You were brilliant," I exclaimed. "How did you know what they were going to do? I had no idea!"

Mary smiled.

"I've had fifteen years in Mental Health," she said.

I felt very unsettled after the grilling in Dr Desa's office and tried my best to avoid him from then on. It must also have been frustrating and embarrassing for him, being bested by two females.

I felt some sympathy for the Chief and his men. If a complaint escaped and made it to the level above them, they effectively received a black mark for poor management. If enough black marks accrued, there would be repercussions—lack of promotion, transfer to a less-desirable job, or, in rare instances, termination of employment altogether.

As time went on, work became tedious. Regulations tightened, encroaching on schedules, vacations, and even our treatment plans. Pat and I began to feel that our professionalism was being threatened.

One day after Pat returned from repat she came in to work with some exciting news—she was getting married! This beautiful lady with the gentle spirit, who was so much fun to work with, would be leaving the company. She was happy and I could not help but be happy for her although, once again, I would be looking for another helper.

Who would take her place? Mary told me that a therapist was being processed from the Netherlands and was destined for Ras Tanura but it would be some months before it was all finalized.

After Pat left, work pressures again began to get on top of me but there was light at the end of the tunnel—it would not be long until the Dutch therapist arrived. And then Mary called.

"I'm sorry," she said. "The girl from the Netherlands has withdrawn her application."

I was devastated. Mary was sympathetic but there were staff shortages everywhere and I could expect no relief from Dhahran. Time crawled on and she called again with a plan. Three students in their final year had to do their final clinical segments before they graduated. We could rotate them through Ras Tanura as well as other units so they could take the load off the therapists.

It sounded good but there was a catch. They would have time off every day for study, to work on their notes and treatment plans, as well as time off every so often for tutorials in Dhahran. My heart sank again. It was a band-aid solution as far as I could see.

"If I have a choice I'd rather wait for a full-time therapist," I said.

But there was no choice. Mary reminded me that everyone was overworked, and I could either accept the students or have nobody at all. Three students went through my unit. I did appreciate the work they did, although they were slow and cautious, as indeed they should have been.

They had assignments to do and Aramco standards to conform to, and their tutor in Dhahran needed them to attend tutorials from time to time, necessitating time off from patient treatments.

One student, Aziz, was insolent. If he had a patient problem and needed help, he challenged everything I told him. He frequently sat in the staff-room chatting to friends on the telephone.

"Are you having an afternoon off?" I asked him one day.

"Yes, why not!" he answered.

By contrast another student, Khalid, was quiet and studious and intensely interested in his work. He drank in everything he could and asked many questions. A quiet chuckle was always hiding in his wispy black beard. I wanted him to take a permanent position in Ras Tanura when he graduated but he regretfully declined, deciding to work closer to his home in Dammam, for the sake of his family.

Khalid did not flaunt his religion, but we soon discovered that he was a *mutawa*. He told Maria that if he saw her outside the clinic, when he was walking with his wife, to please forgive him for not speaking to her. Mutawa do not generally speak to females unrelated to them, except for disciplinary reasons. The mutawa I had seen thus far had been loud and aggressive, but Khalid showed me the kind, gentle side of his religion.

At this time, everyone in the rehabilitation department seemed to be suffering from low morale. Abdalla, the chief supervisor of Rehabilitation, appeared to take every opportunity to crush his subordinates. Even Mary became frustrated and short tempered at times. Finally she resigned, and returned to Canada.

Katrina, the young Australian therapist who had weathered the mutawa attack outside Safeway with me three years previously, took Mary's job. She was level-headed, full of energy and had good rapport with those in charge. Yet, even she had some difficult days.

Abdalla had been an x-ray technician before he'd worked his way up to the top job in Rehabilitation. He had been the one to interview me in Australia, and had seemed like a very pleasant person. Yet he now seemed to take every opportunity to make life difficult for those under him.

I was disappointed that this apparently nice man seemed not only to be indifferent to the needs of the staff under his influence but to actively treat them with contempt. It was to be only a matter of time before he was transferred.

34 - A BURNING QUESTION

"THERE'S A GRAND piano for sale," Rob said one afternoon as we sat together after work. "The ad is up on the board in the mail centre. Did you realize Peter Burg is the one selling the piano?"

I hadn't.

"Really?" I said vaguely, continuing to read the newspaper.

A few moments later Rob spoke again.

"Maybe you should take a look at that piano."

"Mmmm. Maybe," I said.

Another silence then,

"Let's go over and see that piano."

"OK," I said, "It can't hurt, can it."

The Burgs were obviously in the throes of packing but the piano stood in the living room, black, shiny, inviting. I felt a pang. It had always been a dream of mine to own a grand, and Rob knew it.

"The piano was new when we bought it ten years ago," said Peter. "Unfortunately it was dropped on the wharf in Dammam and the soundboard was cracked."

My heart sank. A broken sound board was usually the dell-knell for a piano.

"However," Peter continued, "the piano tuner started off very cautiously, tightening the strings across the sound board by only a minimal amount and every year since then he has tightened them a little more. Finally it's up to full tension—ten tons of pressure across the sound board. He says it is a very stable crack, but even so we've been advised that we can't ask full price for the piano."

"Why do you want to sell it at all?" I asked, numbly. I knew that Peter enjoyed playing the piano as much as I did.

"Well, I want to buy an electronic piano, so I can use the earphones if Rhona doesn't want to be disturbed. An electronic piano is also easier to transport."

I nodded. Peter was a good pianist. I'd heard him playing a couple of times when he thought no one was listening, but he was rather shy of performing in public.

"Sit down, play something!" said Peter with a smile, "I have to get on with the packing. Take your time."

He left the room. I looked at Rob.

"It's so beautiful!" I whispered.

"Go on, play," he said.

I placed my hands on the keys, noticing the reflections in the black wood behind the keyboard. The first notes of Sibelius' "Romance," rang out in the still room. By the time I'd finished, my knees were shaking.

"I love it!" I said, overcome with dizziness. "I *could* afford this, if I used every riyal I have. If I sold my other piano and used all my savings, I could just do it!"

Rob looked at me strangely.

"You know," he said, "I had always thought I'd like to give you a piano for a wedding present. How about it?"

I gasped. A jolt went through my chest and blood surged though my temples. I couldn't speak but he must have seen the answer in my eyes.

"OK then!" He laughed. "Where would you like to keep it? Your place or mine?"

"Umm, how about your place?" I said at last. "Then it will only have to be moved once."

Peter came back into the room.

"How was it?" he asked. "Are you happy with it?"

"Oh yes!" I said earnestly, unable to keep the smile off my face. "It's absolutely beautiful. I'll...We'll take it. Thank you very much!"

So the piano was mine—and Rob too. I felt as though I'd just been given the world.

"Right, then," said Peter, "you'll need a mover. I could ask the fellows packing for us if they'd like a job on the side, if you want. In their spare time, you know. Their company needn't know about it so we could negotiate a special rate."

"Sounds like a plan," said Rob, "Let's do it."

I placed my old piano in our charity group's annual auction and it raised over twice as much as I'd paid for it. The money from the auction went to help a hospital in Yemen, and to support female Third Country Nationals in Saudi Arabian jails. The new piano was a good trade in every way!

Now—what about the wedding? Should we tell the company that we were getting married? Single women working for Aramco were required to end their contracts if they married so many a couple chose to keep their nuptials secret. There were a certain number of positions for "casual employees," or married women, but there was no guarantee that I'd be offered a job. We decided to lie low for a while and ask a few questions before going public with our plans.

My parents were torn between being pleased for us and shocked by the sudden proposal at my grand old age of forty-one. There were only eight weeks left before repat, and so they were landed with the job of organizing the whole wedding.

"Keep it as simple as possible," I told them. "We're not having any attendants so that should help."

We went to the gold souks in Rahima and I settled on a small gold ring with an indented pattern, but shook my head when Rob asked if I wanted a diamond.

"It's not *me*," I said. The piano is enough; I don't want an expensive stone on my hand as well."

"What about your wedding dress?" my mother wanted to know.

"Oh, I'll pick something up in Brisbane during the week before the wedding," I said airily.

"You will *not!*" She gasped. "You'll have to get something well before that."

Khobar offered nothing to suit a westerner's taste in wedding gowns. I drew the line at frothy, beaded creations with yards and yards of tulle, lace and glitter. There'll surely be something in the new Rashid mall, I thought. In one of the wedding stores.

"Yes!" said a young Indian triumphantly, "We have wedding dresses."

He beckoned conspiratorially as he approached a door to an inner room of the shop. Then he paused at a sudden thought.

"Do you mean a dress for the night or a dress for the party?"

"A dress for the party," I said.

"Oh," he said, disappointed. "I only have dresses for the night."

I never did see the seductive little numbers that were tucked away beyond the gaze of disapproving mutawas.

"We'll have to *make* the dress," said my mother, who had walked the streets of Brisbane with her cousin, Barbara, and found no wedding dresses suitable for a skinny and elderly spinster.

"All the ready-made dresses are off the shoulder," she said. "There's nothing here that you'd like."

One of the benefits in Aramco was access to an excellent library including pattern catalogues, which passed unscathed through Saudi Arabian censorship. I pored over the bridal sections in these catalogues until I found The Dress.

My mother's cousin, Barbara, would make it. She was a professional seamstress and by a strange coincidence the pattern I had chosen was the same pattern she had used for her own wedding dress a few years earlier. The design was simple. It was not "fussy", and hung elegantly.

We'd be in Australia for just a week, and decided that the wedding should be on a Friday. It so happened to be the Fourth of July—American Independence Day.

"Odd, isn't it, that we should lose our independence on Independence Day," said Rob.

There was no way I could match the splendor of a grand piano, when choosing a wedding gift for Rob. He enjoyed Saudi Arabian antiques but he had samples of most Middle Eastern artifacts. Except a Saudi Arabian sword.

I found one in an antique store on King Khalid Street in Khobar. It was long, heavy and encased in a sheath of silver filigree.

"Has it cut any heads?" I asked the shopkeeper.

He smiled.

"Four or five," he joked.

"Will it cut one more?" I asked.

"Sure it will!"

Exactly a month before the wedding, my father called from Australia.

"Honey," he said. "Forget the wedding; it isn't going to happen."

My heart skipped a beat.

"What do you mean?"

"Well, I asked you to send the documents the minister asked for. They have to be here a month before the wedding day. You said you'd sent them but—well, they haven't arrived and today is the last day. I don't know what else to tell you."

"But I sent them by courier a week ago!" I said wildly. "They told me they'd arrive in three days! They *can't* be lost. We can't postpone the wedding; we've made all the bookings and the repat dates can't be changed..."

"Hold on a minute," Dad said.

There seemed to be some kind of commotion before he came back on the line. I could hear the smile in his voice when he spoke.

"It's OK! The delivery van just arrived and your mother has the documents in her hand right now. We'll drive over to the minister's house immediately!"

I fell into the chair behind me and allowed the tension to drain from my body.

"Whew! That was a close call."

And so, with the arrangements for the wedding under control, we lived our last few weeks of single life.

35 - HARD PRESSED

IT HAD BEEN a particularly busy morning and Hamad had come in late for his appointment anyway. I had set him up with a hot pack on his knees while I attended to other patients—and completely forgot about him. I'd just finished lunch by the time the horrible truth dawned on me.

"Hamad!" I gasped as I flew out to the work area.

At the same instant I flung open the curtains, Hamad woke up and realized that his hot packs were cold. We stared at each other in shock.

"I'm so sorry!" I said. "I'll take those off you and finish your treatment."

"You forgot me!" he shouted. "That is not good!"

"You're right, that's not good, and I am very sorry. Now, will you let me finish your treatment?"

Hamad launched into a tirade. I had forgotten him, I was not a good person and he did not appreciate the treatment, or lack of, that I had given him.

"...so you throw me as you would throw a ring from your finger!" he concluded.

"I said I am sorry," I pleaded. "What more can I do?"

He stomped out in disgust and called the department office in Dhahran, as I feared he might do.

"What did you do to him?" Maria asked, mystified.

"I forgot him," I said glumly.

"You *forgot* him?" she repeated incredulously.

"Yes. Well, I was very busy that morning but I know that's no excuse. I just forgot about him!"

She sighed sympathetically.

"Well, he doesn't want you to continue his treatments but he's condescended to see Suheim. I suggest you tell Suheim what you want done with him and have Suheim check with you on treatment progression. Good luck!"

I breathed a sigh of relief. I was not going to be chastised or given my marching orders but I scolded myself furiously for the mistake, and ever after checked every cubicle repeatedly.

It was bound to have happened sooner or later. I was so busy that my patients frequently had to wait for my attention during the course of a treatment, and it was becoming harder and harder to juggle appointments.

Suheim was working in Dhahran by now, but had come up to relieve Zahara who was on vacation. I was proud of the way he carried off Hamad's treatments. He liaised with me at every step and mollified Hamad in his own special way. Truly that young man could pour oil on troubled waters better than anyone I have ever known.

I generally had good rapport with the physicians in the clinic, but I noticed that many of them did not refer patients in the acute stages of their problem, but waited until the patient was chronic before sending them in to me. This bothered me. Physical Therapists like to see patients as soon as possible after the onset of their symptoms as results are usually quicker and patients don't need as many treatments. I thought that if only I could persuade doctors to send me patients when they were acute, as time went on my workload would be less.

One doctor in particular seemed to delay his referrals beyond the appropriate time. It was Dr Ibn Aljam, the deputy liaison officer for the clinics, who had given me such a hard time at the meeting in the CEO's office. I made an appointment to see him.

"Hello," I said, pulling up a chair. "I just wanted to chat for a couple of minutes about referrals."

"Yes?" he said with a cursory nod of the head.

"Well, I've noticed that some of the physicians don't refer to me until the patient has had several visits with them. I just thought that if you could...er...encourage them to refer patients earlier, say when they were first diagnosed with their complaint, we might be able to deal with their problems more quickly and solve the problem before it develops into a *big* problem."

"What do you mean?"

"Back patients, for example, especially do well if they can be seen as soon as possible after injury. If we do not see them quickly, they can take much longer to treat, or could even worsen to a point where therapy is of no use. I would really like the spinal patients to be referred immediately if possible."

Ibn Aljam fixed a beady eye on me.

"I don't understand why you have to see back patients early," he said. "I can evaluate them and treat them in my office. I don't usually need to send them to you."

"Well if I were to see them early, perhaps they would only need one or two treatments," I said calmly. "If they are referred some weeks after first presenting, they may need to have several weeks of treatments."

"I can evaluate a patient in five minutes and give him exercises. Why should it take you so long?"

I smiled.

"It just takes time to educate the patient and involve him with a treatment program. Anyway, thanks very much for your time. I must get back to my work now."

It had been a useless exercise. I turned my thoughts to something else that needed attention—the window in our reception room. Patients could not be heard or make themselves heard unless both parties pressed their ears up against the window, for sound did not carry well through the tiny 'communication' holes in the partition.

Trying to make appointments and do other business was sometimes so difficult that we would bring the patient into the reception room so we could hear each other.

In vain I had asked for someone to look at it and either enlarge the holes or replace the glass with a window which could slide back. Maintenance was reluctant for us to use an open window, as they suspected people could reach in and take things from the desk when the receptionist's back was turned. I wrote another referral for evaluation of the window.

At about this time we received a call from Dhahran to inform us that an appraisal team was coming from the USA to inspect the hospitals and clinics for accreditation. The place was abuzz with activity. The team would spend most of its time in Dhahran, but the satellite clinics would also be inspected, and we were instructed in what to say and do. It was comforting to know that as our procedures were identical to those in our Dhahran unit we were not directly in the firing line.

The big day came, and a memo arrived from Dr Samudra, who was the physician selected to introduce the team. It informed us that he and the team would be calling on our unit after lunch at around twelve thirty pm. We were ready. Time ticked on. Two o'clock, two-thirty, three o'clock. I was puzzled. Surely they should have been here by now.

The other clinics in Ras Tanura opened at seven in the morning, closed for an hour over lunch and everyone went home at four in the afternoon. Our hours were the same as those of the rehabilitation unit in Dhahran, for ease of operations—we opened at seven in the morning, closed for only half an hour for lunch, and locked up at three thirty in the afternoon unless I was running late, which was often the case.

We had blocked off some time for the inspection and some of the scheduled patients did not show, so this afternoon we managed to finish on time. I sent Suheim home.

"I'll just tidy up," I said. "I guess the team isn't coming now."

At twenty minutes to four I switched the lights off in reception. Glancing through the window I spotted Dr Samudra.

"Hello!" I called. "Are you here with the accreditation team?"

He said something through the reception window which I did not hear, naturally.

"This is a late twelve thirty!" I said, gesturing to the door. "Come on in."

Nobody opened the door, and so I did. Dr Samudra came in, obviously flustered. Two Americans followed him. We introduced ourselves.

"Sorry about this, but we're just finished for the day," I said. "I'd be happy to show you through the unit though. What would you like to see?"

They walked quickly around our small room, asked a few questions and went on their way.

"Enjoy the rest of your time in Saudi Arabia," I said as they left.

A week later I had a call from Gordon Gambel, who had been appointed above Mary as yet another supervisor. I had heard that Gordon could be very tough on his subordinates, but he had always been civil to me and I meant to keep it that way. All the same, I was a little perturbed that he wanted to see me.

When I arrived, Gordon was pleasant. We chatted for a few moments before he got down to business.

"I've had a complaint about you," he said, looking at me over the top of his glasses.

"Really?" I asked, palpitations surging again in my chest.

"Yes," he said. "Listen while I read you a letter."

He leaned back in his chair, rested his right elbow on the table and shuffled some papers. As he read, my blood froze.

Dr Samudra had written a long and detailed dissertation on the accreditation visit, complaining about me *locking the unit door* on the visiting team from the USA so they could not enter for their inspection! By the time he had finished I was writhing.

"Oh, Gordon!" I said, "I had no idea he was upset. I've always liked him and gotten on well with him. I'd hate for this to come between us."

I explained the problem we had with our window, and told the story from my point of view.

"He must have misunderstood me through that window," I concluded. "And at no time did I *ever* lock anyone out!"

Gordon looked at me sympathetically.

"He probably didn't realize that your unit closes at three thirty, whereas the RT clinics all close at four.

I suggest you write to him," he said. "You need to explain what happened."

I nodded, feeling numb and sick at the same time.

"He must have felt so embarrassed in front of the visitors," I said. "I will write to him. I'll apologize for any misunderstandings and we will really have to get that window changed!"

I wrote a heartfelt apology to Dr Samudra, and copied it to Gordon. There was no response from Dr Samudra to my message, but the next time I met him he was as warm and friendly as ever. Relieved, I realized the matter had been swept away. And not long afterwards, our reception window was replaced with a more communication-friendly one.

36 - TO HAVE OR TO WITH-HOLD?

BLACK BLOBS AND white patches featured in almost every magazine sold in Saudi Arabia. Bands of serious men armed with black felt pens and little pieces of sticky white paper worked their way through everything that entered the Kingdom.

Anything that might corrupt the morals or titillate the passions was scribbled on or covered over. Ads for alcoholic drinks, skin exposed by low necklines and high hems, and pictures of men and women in close contact were censored out.

It was not only public magazines that were tampered with. Movie-goers on Aramco compounds (where the only movie theatres in Kingdom existed) often found themselves wondering what the heck was going on between clips, and the company's newsletters were carefully screened to ensure that no pictures of men and women standing together were published, unless they were married to each other.

Even the comic strips in the newspaper were doctored. It became a game to guess what had been the original intent of the artist. Sometimes a word would be changed. "Ham and eggs," became "fish and eggs." The dog in the cartoon, "Sergeant Preston," became "Kin," rather than "King," out of respect for the reigning Saudi Arabian monarch.

There was always an "Amazing Facts," cartoon in the back of the Arab News. One day it featured a woman with two artificial legs, who had achieved a record in the tennis world. The artificial legs were blacked out on the cartoon drawing, so as to cover their nakedness.

Once a week a column called "Islam in Perspective" appeared in the Arab News. Questions about religion and social issues were answered here and it taught me a lot about my Arab neighbors and their beliefs. Foreigners often have a distorted view of Islam and its demands on people. Much of the information I'd been given was debunked here.

Questions ranged from things like, "Is it permissible to kill an infidel for no reason?" to "I just got married and discovered that my new wife dyes her hair. Should I divorce her?" The answers were usually lengthy. Even though some of the questions seemed trivial, I was strangely touched by the depths at which religion reached into the lives of the people around me.

When returning from my first repat, I packed with care, as the customs officials were thorough in their checks. As well as alcohol, drugs and anything smacking of pornography, materials which could be considered anti-Islamic (such as books and papers promoting other religions, and a whole host of items produced by banned organizations) were also *'haraam'* or forbidden.

Everything produced by Israel, or Jewish companies, was banned, and electronic gadgets such as two-way radios and tracking devices were prohibited under the guise of 'National Security'.

I had been trying to create some interesting non-alcoholic drinks for my guests on the compound, but much as I looked I could find no bitters or Grenadine to use as seasonings. So, on my first repat I brought some in, along with the special lime cordial I had loved in my home country. The labels were all clear of any suspicious products as far as I could make out. I'd also bought several videos.

"Anything to declare?" asked the customs official at Dhahran airport.

"I only have these drinks and a few videos," I said happily, putting the bottles and tapes up on the counter. "See? No alcohol!"

The officer gave the bottles a quick glance before waving dismissively.

The videos were quite another matter though. I sat in the office of the head customs official for some time, discussing the content of the videos. All were rated 'G,' except for a set of the "Anne of Green Gables," videos which were rated 'PGR'. The official pointed this out.

"I have no idea why that rating is on there!" I said, mystified. "These are children's stories, pictures for girls. There is nothing bad on these films."

The official had already seen "Beethoven," "Sister Act," and "The little Princess," and I had the feeling he would like to see "Anne of Green Gables," too.

"Where do you live?" he asked.

"Ras Tanura."

I knew that usually videos had to be left for the officials to view and censor and my heart sank. It was very late at night and it was a long way home. To come back to the airport later on would be a major undertaking—an expensive taxi ride (for I couldn't expect a male friend to take time off to bring me all the way down here again) and time off work.

The official must have seen the fatigue in my eyes, and compassion kicked in.

"Take them," he said.

I thanked him fervently and, gathering up my loot, trundled out to get a taxi. More than a little rivalry went on between the taxi companies. Two major companies held contracts for delivering passengers to and from the airport—the yellow cabs and the white cabs.

The yellow cabs were usually rather knocked about; the drivers were not always careful and were sometimes downright dangerous. The smart-looking white cabs, on the other hand, were air-conditioned, and driven at respectable speeds by drivers who handled their charges with care.

The white cabs had the contract to take all Dhahran passengers from the airport so expats from that compound had no worries. However all other passengers, including those from Ras Tanura, were supposed to take yellow cabs.

I had learned how to get a white cab anyway. Going to the white cab stand, I slid a piece of paper, on which was written "Ras Tanura," across the desk.

Nothing was spoken, in case a yellow cab driver happened to be within earshot.

Outside, the white cab driver loaded up my luggage and drove a few minutes down the road to the depot. Then he quickly switched my luggage to an unmarked van and headed up the highway to Ras Tanura. This little routine was always successful.

It was not until the next day, when talking to friends about my purchases, that I discovered a horrible truth—I had brought an alcoholic beverage into Saudi Arabia! There, in bold vertical type on the bottle of bitters, which I had been so proud of and worked so hard to find, was the declaration, '41% alcohol'. My innocence and openness had impressed the customs official so much that he hadn't bothered to check the bottles for himself.

Rob and I bought a new GPS on what turned out to be our last repat. We needed it to facilitate our desert wanderings, so felt justified in smuggling it into the country. On that last repat we also boldly brought in a metal detector and two-way radios.

The night before we left the USA with our treasures, we disguised the items as much as we could. Detachable aerials were removed and packed in other bags and animal stickers were plastered over the equipment to encourage the idea that they were kids' toys.

When the customs officer in Jeddah opened a duffel bag, the first item to fall out was the large head for the metal detector. *Oh no! Why didn't we pack it a bit deeper?*

"What's this?" asked the officer.

"Ummm, electronic drum," I said, with a pang of guilt.

Friends over the years have shared some interesting stories about Customs. A black American friend brought a Michael Jackson CD from the USA one year.

"*Haraam!* Forbidden!" said the customs officer.

"No way!" said our friend.

"I have to take it."

She stared at him suspiciously.

"What will you do with it after you take it?"

"I will put it into this drawer, and when I get enough of them I will burn them."

"In that case, give it to me and I'll break it now."

"No! No! It won't break!"

"Yes it will. Give it to me and I'll break it now."

She took the CD out of his hand and broke it. She says there were tears in his eyes.

On another occasion a dependent wife saw an article, which her friend had ordered from the US, for sale in a shop window in Khobar. The item was still in its box and the woman recognized the name of her friend printed on the outside of the box along with the badge number. She called her friend, who came immediately to Khobar to meet her.

The two women found a mutawa on the street and explained the situation to him. He went into the shop and demanded that the shop owner give the item up to its rightful owner. Mutawas, I decided, have their uses after all.

37 - AN ANCIENT LAND

NORTH OF RIYADH lie the fertile plains of the Al Jawf region, where the earliest signs of habitation in Saudi Arabia can be found. This was on our list of must-see places. The Arabian Natural History Association planned a visit to this area the month before our wedding and Rob and I were eager to sign up.

To my delight Tanya and some of the other single girls had decided to make this trip too, as had some single men. One of the latter was Russel, a tall and handsome black American, a dermatologist recently employed by the company. That evening we all sat together over a buffet with salads, meats, and Middle Eastern delicacies while our leader, Dane Tesach, briefed us on the planned activities for the week.

A Saudi Arabian archaeologist would be available to accompany us to several of the historic sites and answer questions, and a large Mercedes bus would provide transport in comfort. All meals would be provided. We spent a day flying to Riyadh and on to Sakaka, where our group was met and driven by bus to the hotel.

"Can you believe this?" I exclaimed as we entered the reception area. "It's like an exotic Spanish villa!"

We walked through terracotta arches and Bougainvillea-lined pathways to our rooms. Air-conditioned and supplied with every convenience, it was a far cry from the homes of the Bedouin just a few miles away.

It was a land of contrasts. From a residence of modern luxury we launched out into the world of antiquities. A gigantic well from the time of the Nabateans supplied a sophisticated irrigation system which is still in use today, providing farm land with precious water. Nearby stood the rocky ruins of Qasa Marad, a fortress dating to 2000 BC, where ancient rock art abounds in several areas. Then there was Rajajil, the Saudi Arabian equivalent of Stonehenge, believed to be over five thousand years old.

Non-Moslems are allowed to enter the Mosque of Omar, the oldest mosque in Arabia still in use. Here rich red prayer rugs contrast with stone pillars and the doors, heavily decorated on both sides. Our cameras snapped constantly.

On our last day a visit to a special area in the desert had been scheduled, to an area where the oldest stone implements in the country had been found. The tarmac gave way to a gravel track, which became rougher as we progressed. Suddenly the bus stopped.

"I don't want to go any further," complained the driver. "If we get a flat tire in here I can't fix it and there is no way we can get out."

Dane had a hurried conference with the hotel staff. They were embarrassed; it was the largest group they had ever hosted and they had never used such a big bus before. They decided to scout around a couple of local villages and try to hire any smaller vehicles that were available. Soon a motley collection of vans and pickups arrived and we scrambled aboard.

When we finally climbed out onto hot, hard, ground, a field of rocks lay before us as far as we could see. The archaeologist pointed out axes, chisels, arrowheads and grinding stones and explained their uses before encouraging us to look for some on our own. The older the tool, the more difficult it was to identify, as its construction was more primitive. Of course the pieces we collected had to be left behind as it was an historic site.

Finally it was time to go. I climbed into an air-conditioned van with Tanya and several other girls, while Rob got into the back of one of the pickups. Somebody fastened the tailgate and off they went ahead of us. We chatted as we rode.

"Look!" Tanya exclaimed all of a sudden. "Something's fallen out of the truck in front. It looks like a bundle of old clothes. Oh...it's Rob!"

No! Our van pulled up and I vaguely remember pushing someone out of the way and sprinting to where Rob lay unconscious on the track. Russel was there ahead of me, taking Rob's pulse.

Rob's head was bleeding. His face was very pale. His breathing was fast and deep as though he'd been running and I forced away thoughts of a long rehabilitation.

It was several minutes before he stirred. His eyes opened but without recognition.

"What happened?" he asked through one side of his mouth.

"You fell off the truck and hit your head," I said, trying to remain calm.

He could squeeze my hand with his right hand and then the left and move each leg in turn. Nothing seemed to be broken but Russel discovered a large egg on the back of Rob's head and a couple of nasty grazes on his upper back. Rob stared blankly at me, uncomprehending.

"What happened?" he asked again. The left side of his face remained flaccid.

Now everyone was crowding around, wanting to see if Rob was alright. Russel decided that Rob was fit enough to travel back to the hotel but wanted him to lie flat in the back of the pickup. Once back at the bus he could sit up. On the way he continued to ask what had happened to him, and then threw up. Fortunately we had a plastic bag handy.

We were due to catch the plane out that afternoon. Should we take Rob with the group or look for a doctor here? The local clinic was closed for prayer. Russel thought quickly.

If we waited too long we'd miss the plane. Even if we got an x-ray there was little that could be done out here and there would be no more flights out until tomorrow. If Rob needed decompression surgery he would have to be near a hospital. He'd have to fly back with us.

Dane sidled up to me.

"Err, I hate to say this Judy, but the hotel people feel responsible because they asked the locals to lend their truck. They are afraid the police will be involved. If it's known to be a road accident the driver will be put in jail for at least three weeks until it's all sorted out. Do you...I mean...could you possibly talk to them and give them some reassurance?"

I was shocked. Until now I hadn't thought about the hotel staff or the driver, but we all knew the implications of a road accident.

"Of course!" I said. "It was totally an accident. There is no way that anybody was responsible."

The hotel staff were standing around in the lobby, looking glum.

"Thank you for all you have done," I said. "It most certainly was no fault of yours or of the driver that this happened. It was an *accident!*"

When I told them we would not mention the vehicle involvement when we checked Rob in at the hospital, they were immeasurably relieved.

It seemed like forever until we landed in Dhahran. By this time Bob's memory had improved but he was unable to remember actually falling from the truck. Russel took him to the Aramco hospital.

"I fell from a wall and hit my head on a rock," Rob told the staff.

The police would not be involved, and there would be no delay getting treatment.

When Rob was discharged from the hospital, he was told he should be monitored for a further twelve hours in case of a bleed in the brain.

Russel kept Rob at his own apartment overnight, checked on him several times throughout the night and kept him in the waiting room of his own clinic the next day to make sure he was alright. I was touched; Russel was as fatigued as the rest of us after the long trip.

When our respective families heard about the accident, jokes flew around the world. My family wondered why I was marrying someone who had fallen off the back of a truck. His family, on the other hand, wanted to know if he'd decided to get married before or after the bump on the head.

Dear Tanya, who had been the only other one on the trip to know of our impeding marriage, confessed to me later that, as Rob lay unconscious on the ground, she looked up to the heavens and said fiercely, "They're getting married in a month. Don't You dare!"

Rob returned to Ras Tanura with instructions to rest up a few days. But it was not long before his Scottish heritage rebelled.

38 - BLACK THURSDAY

BORED AT HOME, Rob decided to go to work again three days after his accident. It was too soon. A splitting headache built up as he worked. Thursday morning when I went to see him, he was throwing up again.

I crossed the road to Peter Burg's house and knocked on the door.

"Would you come and see Rob please?" I pleaded. "I'm worried he might have a bleed in his brain."

Peter decided that there was no immediate danger but scolded Rob for going back to work too soon.

"You need to *rest!*" he said. "The fact that you were knocked out for a period of time means that your brain was concussed, or bruised, and you need plenty of sleep and no exertion. You will feel tired for quite some time."

Relieved, I left the patient resting in bed while I dealt with his kitchen. Pest Control was coming to do the final spray for cockroaches after the weekend and everything had to be taken out of his cupboards and piled into the lounge room. There was no way Rob could manage it in the state he was in. And in a few hours' time the movers would be arriving with my piano.

I marveled at the amount of food crammed into Rob's cupboards. Every shelf was in a state of chaos. This would be a good opportunity to reorganize. The pile of tins and packets on the lounge room floor had grown to an alarming height when a commotion sounded at the door. The bell rang several times; someone was shouting my name. I rushed out. Sri, my Sri Lankan houseboy was there, breathless from hurrying.

"Come quickly! Your house...a pipe broken, water...everywhere running...downstairs..."

He took off on his bicycle with me in hot pursuit on mine. I bounded through the doorway into ankle-deep water. It flowed from the ceiling and down the sodden passageway, seeking its level on the lower floor. Upstairs, a rod of water hammered across the tiny bathroom. A pipe behind the toilet had rusted and finally blown out.

"Quickly!" I cried. "Turn the water off!"

"I can't find the main tap!" Sri squeaked.

I rushed about aimlessly looking for it, feeling foolish that I knew so little about the plumbing. Hands trembling I picked up the phone and punched in the number for Maintenance.

"Please hurry," I implored. "This is an emergency! I can't find the tap for the water main."

I was sure the water supply for a week in the whole camp had passed through my apartment by the time the men arrived, turned off the water and assessed the damage.

"We'll have to take the carpet out of the hallway downstairs and dry it out," they said.

I would have to use the bathroom downstairs until this one was fixed and they would arrange to replace the downstairs ceiling and to repaint. I groaned. It was going to mean a lot of time off work. Maintenance men would not come while the place was unattended, for security reasons. Then I glanced at my watch. The piano movers! They'd be at Rob's any second.

"I have to go," I said. "Thank you very much for your help."

Rob was asleep again when I checked on him. By the time the doorbell rang I had a place ready for the piano. The young Pakistanis had the huge instrument on a low trolley; they sweated as they heaved it sideways through the door and eased it down the passageway to the lounge room.

Before long the piano stood proudly on its three legs again, glistening in the late afternoon light. I paused for a moment, overcome by its magnificence, and reflected.

The troubles of the day seemed to vanish. This was more than just a musical instrument—it was a symbol of love. I touched its black sheen reverently with one finger. Then I lifted the lid and began to play. Everything was going to be all right.

39 - TYING THE KNOT, AUSSIE STYLE

WE HAD BOOKED the dates for our repat and worked the wedding into the first week of it. Then we turned our attention to Hobie, the cat. The thought of leaving him alone for five weeks worried me and we decided that it might be a good time to find a permanent home for him.

Then we heard that Gary, the supervisor of the dental clinic, had just lost a cat and was looking for another one. I called him immediately and he was delighted to take the beautiful cat.

"We'll bring him over," I said. "I'll borrow a kennel."

Before Hobie knew what had happened he was locked up and in the car. His sorrowful Siamese yowling broke my heart.

"It's alright!" I reassured him. "You're going to a beautiful new home and Gary will love you to bits."

"I'll keep him indoors for a couple of weeks," Gary promised. "When I'm sure he has adjusted I'll give him some freedom."

"Great," I said. "It's a huge relief to know that we don't have to worry about the cat anymore."

We considered again the difficult question—should we tell Aramco we were getting married? If we didn't and the company discovered we were married I would probably lose my benefits. I also didn't want to have to live a lie. A few questions to Maria assured me that a casual position would probably be on offer if I married. OK, we'd make it official! Our delighted friends wished us well as we set off for the long flight to Australia.

"We're bumping you up to business class," said the air hostess as we climbed the stairs to the waiting area in Bahrain airport.

We grinned at each other. The flight to Singapore was very comfortable, in spite of the fact that we were not seated together. When the evening meal arrived, a small red rose lay beside each plate. I raised mine to my nose and took a sniff. A second rose arrived by my plate—I looked up in surprise. Rob was smiling down at me.

"Never say I don't give you flowers!" he joked.

Rob's mother, Nora, was waiting for us, along with my parents, at the airport in Brisbane.

"I can't believe how cold it is here," she said. "It's colder in the house than it is outside!"

"Winter is so short here that people don't bother with central heating the way they do in Canada," I told her. "We just wear more clothing until it warms up again."

I was touched by how much effort my parents had put into making our wedding day special.

"We've tried to give small companies as much business as possible," my mother said. "The photographer is a friend whose daughter is a professional photographer—they'll do the photos together. The flowers have been ordered and the programs came back from the printer yesterday.

"The church you wanted in the middle of Brisbane was available but everyone says it would be too hard to get parking there during the week and the traffic would be very noisy. So we've booked a pretty little white church in Graceville—lucky it's a Friday wedding because most churches are booked up months, even years, in advance for weekends.

"And everyone getting married these days has to have premarital counseling sessions so we've made some appointments for you with the minister. We've been running around like crazy for the past eight weeks! Oh—you have to have a couple of dress fittings with Barbara this week too."

"We should have gotten married in Bahrain," said Rob. "It would have been much easier. Cheaper too."

"No!" said my mother, "You've made the right decision. Better to be married at home so all the family can attend."

I was curious to see The Dress. My inclination had been for a simple, flowing dress which wasn't a typical 'wedding dress,' but something classically elegant.

The Dress had a mandarin collar, tapered waist, handkerchief hems, and full sleeves with long cuffs. Buttons and loops closed the cuffs and the back opening. It was all-over lace. It *was* a 'real wedding dress'. But I loved it!

"It's just about finished except for the side seams," said Barbara. "I wanted to make sure it was a perfect fit before the final stitching."

She decided to sew some tiny pearls around the skirt, emphasizing the lower bodice edge, and used the last piece of fabric to make a small bag which would hang from my wrist and hold a handkerchief.

Although I loved my wedding dress, I was beginning to feel uneasy about it all. I'd never liked being the centre of attention. Fuss had always made me nervous and as the big day came closer both Rob and I became more uncomfortable.

"We could have gotten married in Bahrain," said Rob. "It would have been much easier than this."

"Quiet! Please!" my mother said.

Rob and I took his mother to Brisbane's South Bank the day before the wedding. It was relaxing, walking around the fountains and the art gallery, looking at the site of Expo '88 at Southbank and across the river to the city. We had lunch at the Ned Kelly restaurant and visited the animal park, where a koala escaped from the pen and went sprinting down the walkway.

"I didn't know they could move so fast," Rob remarked.

He pointed out the escapee to a ranger who went in pursuit of the errant animal.

"That's the third time this week he's done this," grumbled the ranger as he returned with the miscreant under his arm. The little animal's face was a picture of resignation.

Then a sign in the park caught my attention.

"There's a ballet here tonight," I said. "The Queensland Ballet company is performing 'Sleeping Beauty'."

We were all interested, so I called home.

"We'd like to go to the ballet down here tonight," I said to my mother. "Is there any reason why we need to come home early?"

"You can't go to the ballet!" my mother exclaimed.

"Why not?"

"It's the night before your wedding! And you have your final dress fitting tonight!"

"All right," I sighed. "We'll come home."

"We could have gotten married in Bahrain you know," Rob said again, that night over dinner. "It would have been a lot easier!"

40 - CASUAL OR CASUALTY?

RAIN WAS FORECAST for the fourth of July, but the day dawned cloudless and sunny. Although the weather was beautiful and the wedding itself turned out to be one of the most memorable experiences of my life, I felt fractured somehow—it seemed we had cheated our friends in Arabia. Perhaps we really *should* have been married in Bahrain! Or at least had some kind of celebratory function there.

Both Rob and I had dreaded the arrival of the wedding day, but to our surprise found the day a pleasure. The little white church seemed a perfect venue, and the officiating minister ended the simple church service by wrapping a cord around our clasped hands, "tying the knot," in an ancient tradition.

The reception was in a nearby town, and was equally delightful. There was a minimum of fuss and some said it was the loveliest wedding they had ever attended.

We had our honeymoon in Vanuatu. It was not a random choice. The island nation was a potential residence after Aramco and we needed to investigate the possibilities further. Rob booked five days at a hotel in Port Vila on the main island of Efate and two in Luganville on the large island of Santo.

We snorkeled, hiked, ate wonderful food, toured the islands and enjoyed beautiful sunsets. It seemed almost like coming home for me as I'd grown up in Polynesia. It would not take much effort to adapt to life here, I thought.

After a week in Vanuatu we flew to Sydney where we met my parents and Nora, who'd all driven down from Brisbane while we'd been away. A couple of days later we flew back to North America, with Nora. The next few weeks involved long drives around beautiful Nova Scotia and spending time with Rob's family in Canada.

We arrived back in Saudi Arabia in the early hours one Sunday morning. As we got out of our taxi in front of the house, a cream-and-chocolate cat stalked across the road and sat down with its back to us.

"Oh no!" I cried. "There's Hobie!"

The big Siamese was obviously very cross with us and it was three days before he would allow himself to be petted as normal.

"I kept him in the house for two weeks," Gary told us. "He stayed under the bed the whole time. Finally, I thought I'd open the door to the upstairs balcony so he could enjoy some sunshine but as soon as he got out he was off. He spent the last three weeks over at your place. I put food out for him every day but there was no way I could get near him!"

"I'm so sorry! I guess we're stuck with him," I sighed. "You'll be better off with a young kitten."

The welcome our friends gave us was touching. Maria put on a party for us in Dhahran and I was overwhelmed. She and Dean were truly some of the kindest people I had ever met. She told me that the wheels were turning on an offer for casual employment and that I should continue working as normal until the formal offer was made.

The company paid for a shipment, back to Australia, of things I would not need when I moved in with Rob. My dear husband was a packrat and his house was full. As every available nook and cranny was stuffed with his precious things, there was no room for mine! I spent several days sorting and stacking boxes in his spare room and finally emptied my former apartment.

For the last time I wandered through the rooms of my bachelor apartment. I'd woken up in the bedroom every morning with the sense of being on vacation.

Now the terracotta wall in the kitchen had been restored, with some effort, to its required shade of white. There was the living room where I had played my first piano, which had once annoyed my neighbor so much. The corner where I'd arranged silk poppies and roses in a copper pot. The pantry where the huge rat had met his demise.

My large potted tree had now gone to another home, along with the stereo system and my beautiful oriental rugs. It was time for me to go too. Taking a deep breath, I closed the door behind me and walked away to my new future.

It took some months for the offer of casual employment to come to me and, in the meantime, I continued working. I had promised Maria I would stay on staff in Ras Tanura. We were still awaiting a permanent second staff placement.

The casual offer came like a pot of black paint dumped on white carpet. Abdalla, the infamous Supervisor of Rehabilitation, not only wanted me to continue working for a drop in grade code, but to take a drop to the lowest level of that grade code!

In practical terms it meant a reduction in pay to around a third of what I had been making, with no other benefits. I was astounded. I'd always had the highest performance ratings, always been careful to give my best to the unit and this was the best they could do. I felt sick.

"Don't accept!" everyone in my department begged. "If you do, we'll lose that grade code from your unit and maybe we won't get it back. Negotiate to keep the grade code."

Abdalla treated all the staff under him shabbily and morale was consistently low. I had felt fortunate indeed to be in Ras Tanura, away from his immediate influence, but now it was my turn to writhe under his mean spirit. Three times I went back to the casual employment negotiator.

"I don't mind stepping down from the top job," I said. "Give me the grade ten position and appoint someone else to the grade eleven."

My pleas were ignored and finally the negotiator called me to say, "I'm so sorry, Abdalla has withdrawn the offer of employment."

A flood of emotions filled my veins. My initial reaction was laughter!

"That's fine," I said. "I'm actually very happy about that!"

"Guess what," I told Zahara jubilantly, "I don't have to come to work anymore!"

Zahara looked devastated. She stared at me disbelievingly and I felt ashamed for being so glad.

And I had let Maria down. I'd promised to remain on staff and now she would have to struggle to replace me. I cancelled patients for the rest of the week and finished as many discharge summaries as possible.

Ras Tanura Physical Therapy department got to keep their grade code eleven. They replaced me with Lorraine, a lovely English therapist from Udailiyah, who had been on the cards to transfer to Ras Tanura as the second therapist anyway.

"I was looking forward to coming to Ras Tanura and working with you," she lamented. "Not on my own!"

The sense of freedom was exhilarating when I woke up the next morning and realized that my duties at the clinic were finished for good. About a month later I had to go to the clinic for an appointment. but, as I rounded the last corner, my bike came to a stop seemingly all by itself. There seemed to be an almost physical barrier between me and the building. Don't be silly, I scolded silently, and forced myself to ride on.

It took time to regain my energy after quitting work. I had not realized how much the job had been wearing me down until I left it.

Aramco gave me a handsome severance pay and I was able to complete the mortgage on my house with the lump sum, which gave me immense satisfaction. Although I'd had some problems with the people in my work situation, the company as a whole had been very, very good to me. I never had any regrets about working for Saudi Aramco.

My time was now spent on housework and yard work so Rob and I could have leisure time together when he came home in the afternoons. I could go shopping when I wanted and attend functions with other dependent wives during the day.

My days became so full that I began to wonder how women managed who did all this and had children too. It was not always easy, being a dependent wife. And there was now no pay packet at all.

I enjoyed the sudden and prolonged 'vacation' but was aware that some dependent wives longed for fulfilling employment in jobs unavailable to them. For skilled and intelligent women, the enforced leisure time could be unwelcome.

41 - A SLIP OF THE FINGER

DECEMBER ROLLED ON and our first Christmas as a married couple approached. That year the company sent out memos advising that under no circumstances would any Christmas lights be allowed. And so, at precisely five-thirty the next evening, the sky above Ras Tanura lit up with the blaze of all the Christmas lights on camp.

Rob made plans for his annual Christmas party.

"I've got over two hundred people on the list this year," he said. "I'll try to send as many invitations out by email as possible."

Although Internet was not freely available in the Kingdom as yet, the company offered email facilities and sending invitations this way was a lot easier than printing and mailing bundles of envelopes.

One of the first to respond to the invitation, with regrets, was a Saudi Arab from the gas plant where Rob worked. Rob thought that that was odd since he had not invited him to the party. Each year he invited a few Saudi Arabian friends, people who had lived in the West and enjoyed the company of expatriates, but this man was not amongst them.

Rob checked his emails outbox and discovered, to his chagrin, that he'd emailed his invitation to a 'Thought of the Day' group by mistake! Almost all of the people on this list were Saudi Arabs. Soon one of the more Westernized Saudi Arabs came to talk with Rob.

"One of the Saudi employees is upset with you," he said. "They think you are trying to convert them to Christianity by inviting them to your party. I said Rob wouldn't do a thing like that. I told them it was just a mistake but they don't believe me."

The controversy raged throughout the unit for days. Suddenly Rob got a letter offering him something he had wanted for years—a transfer to another unit. He was jubilant. After being at the gas plant for twelve years, he had often asked for a move but was denied as it was not company policy to release him. This time, it seemed, they were willing to let him go. A simple mistake had resulted in gaining him his freedom.

"If I'd only known it was this easy I'd have done it years ago," he joked.

Rob tried to get a placement in a northern district plant. However it soon became clear that his unit manager, although wanting Rob out of his current job, still wanted him under his control. Rob was given a position in a unit which serviced the gas plant so he could be called back on jobs when his services were needed.

Try as he would, Rob could not get his preferred placement signed off. His mood began to plummet. And the new job was depressing.

"I feel like a glorified electrician," he fumed. "Changing light bulbs, instead of doing something worthwhile."

He was not alone in his frustrations. Morale was low everywhere. And the price of oil had hit an all-time low. All through the company people were being surplused, or given early retirement.

A surplus resulted in a more desirable retirement package when an expat gave up his position when asked. These benefits were especially prized if you were near to retirement—how much better could it get than to enjoy early retirement with an added bonus? There was a huge exodus of expats eager to take advantage of this opportunity to get their Exit Only visa, meaning their retirement from the Kingdom.

Rob offered his name for surplus. The next surplus list did not include his name, so he kept working on, figuring that he had only three more years to go until he was sixty, when the company would retire him automatically anyway.

When work is not satisfying you turn your attention to vacations. And Rob had been planning our next major trip within Kingdom. This trip had loomed in his mind for the past eighteen years as the ultimate challenge in desert driving—a complete crossing of the Rub Al Khali, the largest sand desert in the world.

42 - THE BIGGEST SANDPIT OF ALL

THE DESERT is harsh. Waves of dry sand extend beyond vision, melting into the horizon in a burning haze. Nobody lives here, though Bedouin pass through from time to time during the winter. Scorpions survive along with snakes and certain lizards that revel in the heat.

It can reach a hundred and forty-four degrees Fahrenheit in one of the hottest places on earth—the *Rub' Al Khali,* or Empty Quarter, of Saudi Arabia. With two hundred and fifty thousand square miles of sand, this is the largest continuous body of sand in the world.

In early 2006 eighty-nine environmentalists, geologists and scientists explored the Rub' al Khali, discovering various fossils and meteor rocks as well as thirty-one new plant species and twenty-four bird species which occur in the area. After this expedition they nick-named the desert *Rub' al-Ghali,* the Valuable Quarter!

We decided to cross this desert by four-wheel drive in the winter of 1998. Although the days would still be uncomfortably hot, there would not be the cruel, blistering heat of the summer. Endless discussions went on amongst the four drivers who would risk their vehicles and the lives of those with them in the days ahead.

We were not the first expatriates by any means to take up the challenge of this desert. Bertram Thomas, St John Philby and Wilfred Thesiger traveled in the Rub al Khali in the 1930s and 40s, and many Aramco geologists and engineers have braved its rigors since oil was first discovered here in 1938. The earliest expeditions were carried out by camel trains.

Each crossing is different, depending on the route one chooses and the weather. It would be eight hundred miles between fuel stations, with no marked tracks to follow. We planned to travel from the far northeast corner of the desert to the southwest corner, the longest possible distance.

The four teams consisted of Don and Alanna and their teenage daughter Hanna, Richard and his son Denis, Frank and Fiona, and Rob and me. Don had mechanical skills which would be deeply appreciated in the days ahead.

Lists were drawn and redrawn, maps studied, meal menus planned and calculations made as to how much fuel would be required by each vehicle. It was agreed that the two Toyotas would carry a hundred and thirty-five gallons of gas each while the two Suburbans would carry one hundred and seventy each.

Supplies were determined, including spares for the vehicles. Those preparing meals figured out what was needed and who would carry it, to eliminate doubling up of cooking utensils. Clothing was chosen carefully. Rescue equipment included long nylon tow ropes, shovels, and winches. There was even a body bag, in case the unthinkable happened and one of us did not make it out of the desert alive.

We all had two-way radios and GPS units but would use them sparingly until we entered less populated areas. They were illegal and Saudi Arabian police would have confiscated them if they were discovered. Off road we would make our way using maps and GPS. If for some reason the satellite system failed us, we would fall back upon traditional methods of compass, maps, and celestial navigation to get us out.

We planned to drive south through the eastern province of Saudi Arabia, to a village called *Salwa*, then turn south-west to *Nibek*, also known as *Anbak*. This was the last fuel stop where we could fill our spare tanks for the off-road portion of the trip. The village consisted of little else but four petrol stations. Seemingly its only function is to provide gas for the Bedou and the occasional expatriate who is foolish enough to enter the desert beyond.

Rob and I had made a preliminary run a month previously to find a good campsite, as it would be around midnight when we arrived here. *Nibek* is surrounded by *subkha*—flat, treacherous, marshy ground which can suck your vehicle down to the axles. We needed a precise point to aim for in the dark.

Departure day found us packed and ready to go. As soon as work was over and last-minute items were stowed away into our vehicles, we climbed in and headed for the meeting point where we'd arranged to join up with the vehicles from Dhahran. After a successful rendezvous we depended on recognizing each other's headlights to keep the convoy intact, for we could not risk using the radios until we were into the desert proper. Half an hour before midnight we arrived at Nibek, hoping to fill the tanks and get an early start in the morning—but the fuel stations were all closed!

Our chosen campsite was nearby in a little haven of sandy hillocks amidst the *subkha*, easily found with the track already on our GPS. Rob and I used our swags (Australian bedrolls with built-in mattresses, enclosed in waterproof canvas sheaths) which rolled out in a moment, and wearily we collapsed into them. At the first sign of morning we reluctantly emerged from our warm cocoons and shivered in the sharp dawn air, hurrying to get back to the fuel station.

Every vehicle had its own method of carrying fuel. We had taken out the rear seats of the Land Cruiser and had tied two large plastic industrial barrels, each full of gasoline, in the gap.

At last we were moving again in the right direction, heavy with fuel and very aware of the dangers of the *subkha*. A good gravel track ran south for a while after *Nibek* but soon we had to leave it and head west, through rocky hills and sandy flats.

This part of the journey required skill and endurance and I was glad that Rob was doing the driving. We aimed to sleep in *Ubaila* the first night, the abandoned Aramco compound which I had seen on my first trip to *Hadida*, the meteorite crater.

Soft sand impeded our progress and we found ourselves exhausted and far from our goal at the day's end. Stocks of fuel and food would diminish as we traveled but right now the extra weight was discouraging and downright hazardous. We were forced to make stops for minor repairs including a leaking bung in one of our fuel barrels which Rob sealed with a piece of heavy plastic. Our homemade roof rack and supports began to shift because of the load, and we adjusted and tightened it at every stop. I wondered if it would see us out.

It supported two spare wheels, a vice, sand boards, shovel, a one inch diameter nylon tow rope, a steel tow cable, a jerry can of spare fuel, engine oil, firewood, and water pumps. Our vehicle was the oldest of the three on this trip—the most experienced we liked to think, but perhaps more vulnerable to breakdown.

After the sand we struck a gravel plain where we made good time but after a couple of hours were into dunes with soft sand again. Progress was slow with sometimes all vehicles stuck at once. Then it was out with the shovels to dig and push out one vehicle at a time. Sometimes a vehicle was barely out of the sand when it became bogged again. The one-inch nylon towrope, with eyes spliced into both ends, became a hero. The towing vehicle would accelerate; the rope would stretch and strain and suddenly pop the bogged vehicle out of the sand like a cork.

Taking the lead involved intense concentration, judging the quality of the ground ahead and choosing the easiest path to follow. We rotated the lead position from time to time to avoid unnecessary fatigue on one driver. There had not been as much rain here as we had hoped; early rains would have hardened the sand crust and made it easier to traverse. It was the season in which we could possibly expect a shower, and several threatening storms passed overhead but only a few drops reached us.

Suddenly, we arrived at a hot sulphurous spring. The stench was unpleasant and the water almost too hot to bear, but the chance to wash our bodies and hair was too strong to resist. Happily the stench soon disappeared after our ablutions.

The heavy physical work of pushing and digging vehicles out of the sand was exhausting and depressing and finally we bedded down where we were, all stuck in the sand. I rose early and took my morning walk among the dunes. How vulnerable our tiny party was in this immense sandy ocean!

The next morning, after an hour and a half of digging, pulling, pushing and towing, we decided reluctantly to air down the tires. With the loads so great we had wanted to retain as much pressure as possible. It made a noticeable difference—we bogged down less often.

The sand, however, was still very hard to read and desperation was beginning to set in when someone, who had walked ahead, returned with the report that *Ubaila* was just around the next dune. Jubilation!

After a late lunch stop the more energetic ones walked over the shimmering sand to investigate the points of interest here—a small wrecked plane and an abandoned nuclear reactor.

After *Ubaila*, hard sand and gravel rumbled under our wheels again and we made up time, but forty minutes before sundown the tow rope had to come out again. We made camp that night in a bushy area at the base of low dunes.

A storm snarled around us that night and I woke up after midnight to find my swag half full of sand. In the beam of my flashlight a tuft of hair was all that could be seen in the area where my husband had gone to sleep. It was impossible to rouse him to sensible conversation so, after half an hour of trying to ignore the wind, I crawled into our vehicle where I finally got some sleep.

By the morning the storm had passed, making it easier to prepare breakfast and pack up. My bedding was hard to find. It is no wonder that mapping this desert is so difficult—a sandstorm can swallow almost anything in a short period of time, and can strip the paint off a truck.

At eight-thirty that morning we arrived at a charted well that we had been aiming for. *Bir Firja* stood in an open area with a few low dunes around it. It was a neat looking well, with the recent addition of a high concrete surround at the top of the shaft. Several impressions of children's feet and hands were embedded in the concrete. The well itself had been dug hundreds of years ago and had watered many generations of Bedouin and animals. A hillock, formed by the dung of many animals, had built up around it.

Richard and his son Denis rappelled to the bottom of the well and Don pulled them back up with his electric winch. The well was dry and any artifacts which may have been in it were covered up by sand.

The water table in Saudi Arabia has dropped alarmingly over recent years and it may yet become as precious a commodity as oil.

An old bayonet lay rusting in the sand nearby. Prior to King Abdul Aziz's time the Arabs were fragmented in tribe and in spirit, occasionally skirmishing amongst themselves, and had no national identity. Today's Bedouin are generally peaceful nomadic people.

During the summer they keep to the edges of the desert, but in the winter months they venture into the depths of it, seeking feed for the animals and watering them from the ancient wells.

Although the water table is dropping, many of these wells are still viable and are kept carefully covered. In the past, enemies would sometimes remove the covers of each other's wells to allow the sand to fill them, rendering them useless.

Animals are wealth to the Bedouin and they sell and trade them for supplies at the markets in border towns such as Hofuf. They also trade old copperware, silver Bedouin jewelry and handwork such as woven rugs. They have learned that these artifacts are sought after by the westerners who work for Aramco and other businesses in the towns.

Bedouin children do not routinely attend schools, although the tuition is free and education is encouraged in townships. Nature is their school and knowledge is passed on from generation to generation. The national religion is Islam and a Saudi Arab changes his religion on pain of death. However the Bedouin, though Moslem, bear some of the superstitions of pagan religions.

Their language is a purer form of Arabic than that of the townsfolk, uncorrupted by the colloquialisms that have crept into the more populous areas. They usually tend their own animals as opposed to the townsfolk who hire cheap Pakistani and Indian laborers to do their work.

It was time to make tracks for *Hadida*. There had not been much change in the craters in the four years since I had first seen them. Particles of iron from the meteorite could still be plucked from the sand with a magnet and I collected more of the shiny 'black pearls' which were formed by the tremendous heat when the meteorite struck the sand.

Suddenly other visitors to the crater arrived. They were from Riyadh and we dallied longer than we intended, sharing stories and plans with them. In this moonscape every human being was an instant friend.

An hour after we left the crater our vehicle stopped. There was not a spark of life in the engine. Don came back to investigate, and after forty-five minutes of analysis sourced the problem—a broken wire, easily repaired. "*Alhumdullilah!* Praise God!" we exclaimed, and were on our way again.

Temperatures were getting warmer as we worked our way further southwest and it was quite hot by day, reaching a hundred and four degrees at times. We did not use the air conditioner, so as to conserve fuel, preferring to leave the windows open. Dehydration was to be avoided at all costs and we were careful to drink plenty of water.

We attempted to find the sealed 'I51' route, a road on the line of longitude 51 degrees East which would make for better driving, but were not in luck.

Although it is on some of the old maps and was once used by the Oil Company in their exploration and development, the desert has silently taken this over too and it is no more. Only vestiges of the route, a marker here and there, were visible as we moved south. There was some comfort in knowing that others had once traveled this way.

Finally we made camp at the base of a small dune, weary but happy to check the maps and note our progress after three full days on the track. Brilliant stars almost exploded from the sky in the blackness of that night.

Next morning as I rolled up my swag, a couple of yellow scorpions scrambled out slowly from tiny depressions they had made in the sand under the canvas. They were cold and sluggish and posed no danger to us.

The pressure of time crowded us, but we dared not hurry. On and on over sandy ridges we plowed. Richard was in the lead but suddenly gave a garbled message on the radio—he had unexpectedly struck the first slip face of the trip. Luckily it was a small one but the descent had been a little sudden nevertheless, and young Dick, who was asleep at the time, was quite shaken. The front bumper had impacted on the hard ground at the foot of the dune and the Suburban was now slightly shortened. Fortunately Richard and Dick had both been wearing their seatbelts.

A friend who had made this trip before had given us coordinates for another artesian well where we arrived late morning. Several minutes later he and his group arrived—they were not making a full crossing, just enjoying a few days in the desert. We enjoyed a quick visit, but as we were behind schedule, we dared not loiter in spite of our fatigue.

So much rain had fallen in this area that it was unbelievably green. White dunes contrasted impossibly with fields of waving grass. A little further on the grass disappeared and dunes flattened into little bushy ridges. The day finished with some rough pounding over lumpy ground. *Irqs*, lines of dunes, began to appear, small and irregular.

Evenings could be balmy and beautiful in the desert, or bitterly cold and damp. Sleeping bags were sometimes wet with dew in the mornings. The silence was astounding. I sat by our campfire and bathed in the isolation and the harmony, so far from the seemingly foolish life we lead in "civilization".

The next day was tediously repetitive. The *irqs* were becoming more defined. These solid lines of dunes do not shift with the wind, and further south they become huge stable landmarks, visible from space and charted on maps. We kept track of which *irqs* we were passing between, not wanting to get too close to the Yemeni border. From time to time we stopped to tighten up the roof rack and discuss the route again with the other drivers, trying to keep radio silence.

Don was having trouble with the second-hand Suburban which he'd bought just before the trip. Extra fuel tanks were installed underneath but he discovered that the wire bundles of electrical circuits were overheating due to insufficient insulation and poor ventilation, causing electrical problems. While the rest of us were having lunch he crawled under the truck and worked on the problem. The wind was increasing, blowing sand parallel to the ground, and when he emerged his face was caked with sand.

It became very bumpy between the *irq*s, with many large bushes close together, difficult to negotiate. I wondered how much the vehicles could take and what the effect on the tires would be. It was tedious in four-wheel-drive and we were burning fuel quickly. Then the bushes thinned out and we were grateful to be able to skip along in two-wheel drive for the rest of the afternoon. We made camp in a sandy hollow and slept like the dead.

Day six dawned. Everyone was weary. We had thought to be near the end of the trip at this point with the driving becoming easier between the *irq*s. But the sand was too soft for rapid progress, and the terrain was uneven with slip faces and low bushes.

Our Land Cruiser began to stall and Don stopped to take a look. An hour later the problem was solved—a loose carburetor screw, another easy fix. We could breathe again.

Now the dunes were larger and more unpredictable. Sometimes we had to stop and walk over to an edge to assess the area and occasionally we had to descend a long slip-face. This involved a little strategy. For a successful descent, the ground at the base of the dune on the downwind side had to be flat or gently sloping downwards with little or no vegetation.

One must drive smartly but not too quickly along the upwind side of a dune. The approach must be direct and the vehicle must accelerate gently but without hesitation until the center of gravity is over the edge of the slip-face. Then it can simply coast, nose down, in an avalanche of sand until the wheels touch the ground at the base and roll away.

Sometimes an approach had to be aborted if the sand was too soft on the upwind side. Occasionally the lead vehicle swerved aside wildly as the driver suddenly realized that he was almost upon a slip-face at an angle and must avoid rolling over the edge. Here the radios were invaluable as the following vehicles could not always see the lead vehicle.

We each had attached a small pole and flag to our roof rack so that our companions in front and behind could spot our location even when our vehicle itself was hidden behind a dune. Thin crust on the sand meant that we had to keep our speed up to avoid bogging down in the soft stuff.

Some of us could hear Yemenis on the CB radios now. There had been incidents involving bandits along the border between Saudi Arabia and Yemen and we were again inclined to keep our distance—and radio silence. Don and Alanna had a *saluki* with them, the type of dog known in the desert for speed and stamina. He was a good watch dog and would alert us of any danger at night.

Gravel plains lay ahead beyond the *irqs*. There were large irregular dunes here and cavernous pits at the bases of some of the long slip-faces. If a vehicle became trapped in one of these there would be no escape. Treacherous sand held all of us in its clutches at times.

Finally, we got stuck in sand up to the axles in a low area. The dunes were so close and irregular that we could not be towed out. A towing vehicle had no room to get speed up, and the sand was too soft. One of the Suburbans perched far above us on a firm spot with its winch cable fully extended down to the end of our winch cable, also fully extended. I began to wonder whether we would have to abandon the faithful old Toyota but after two hours of laborious straining we slowly inched up and out onto hard ground.

It was lunchtime before we reached the flat plains below the *irqs* and our spirits rose in proportion to our speed. But our exhilaration was short-lived. Over the next day and a half we struck bad sand traps leading down into what is called the 'triangle' in the far south west of the country.

We had hoped to make the crossing in six days but the morning of day eight saw us still pushing southwest between towering walls of sand. Our minds were continually on the amount of precious fuel left in each tank. If a vehicle ran dry, we had decided that the smaller vehicles could drive out and return, with their tanks and barrels filled, to share with the Suburbans.

As we barreled along we spotted some worked flint and some of our group wanted desperately to stop and *shuf,* or look around for artifacts. The areas in the southwest corner of Arabia are rich in relics of bygone eras. Arrowheads, spear points, grinding stones and the like are found in abundance. It is a thrill to pick up an implement perhaps not seen or touched by another human in several thousand years.

Older implements are primitive and roughly hewn, taking a practiced eye to spot them amongst ordinary rocks, whereas more recent tools are well defined and skillfully fashioned. We could afford the time to look for arrowheads only after we reached the fuel station and were sure we could return to Ras Tanura on time.

I had a birthday during the trip, and was surprised when the ladies came over from one of the other vehicles with a wonderfully original birthday cake. Fiona had brought it frozen, iced it (Hanna had created a small vehicle with a Twix bar!), put candles on it and presented it to me. I was overwhelmed. Then Bob capped it off by giving me a small crystal grand piano.

"Where did you hide that?" I asked.

"Up on the roof rack, inside the spare tire," he said. "Where do you want to keep it now?"

"In exactly the same place!" I replied.

Finally, at ten-thirty in the morning on day eight, we reached the pavement. It seemed strange to drive on a smooth surface once again. The fuel station was only a few miles away and there we regrouped. Richard had the least fuel remaining, with only two gallons of gas in his tank. We had the most fuel remaining, enough to fill Richard's tank!

We had conquered the desert but it had changed us. Over the past days a dream had been realized, characters strengthened, wits sharpened. None of us would ever be the same again.

43 - OOPS!

THE SUN WAS a golden balloon swelling at the horizon. For a moment it rested there, changing shape in the aura of heat and sand dust, before it fell over the edge and vanished.

In its afterglow shone the faintest fingernail of silver crescents which would set the nation rejoicing. Ramadan had ended. Cannons were sounding in the towns across the country and five days of celebration were beginning.

We were partway along the track to *Shaybah*, planning to visit the company's newest oilfield in the southern desert and return by the end of the Eid holiday.

I dug my toes into the coarse red sand, still warm from the day, and treasured the moment. Around us the landscape was fast disappearing into the calm evening. We built a campfire, had dinner, and sat watching the flames until they died into coals.

Morning came silently. The only signs of life were a high-soaring eagle, and large black beetles that scurried frantically around to find cool havens for the day. Rob started running gas into the fuel tank from a drum we carried in the back seat, and while it trickled in we enjoyed a pancake breakfast. We would have to move on soon before the sun's heat became uncomfortable. Even in winter the maximum for the day could be a hundred and five degrees.

We had camped beside a sand dune which separated us from the track we had followed in. The track was only a set of grooves in the sand, kept alive by the occasional convoy of trucks bearing water and supplies to the embryonic community to the south of us. We felt safe traveling on our own because of this traffic. Rescue would come quickly if we needed it.

A distant drone disturbed the silence—the convoy of today was on the move. A few moments later we saw the water tankers coming . However, instead of following the track which ran around the other side of the dune the first driver, with a mischievous grin and a wave, created another track—right beside our campfire!

Gone was the peaceful morning. The next tanker followed...and the next...and the next...until the only visible track was the one beside our camp. The last tanker rolled to a stop and the driver leaned out of the window, puzzled.

"Why did you camp right by the track?"

"It *wasn't* the track last night when we camped," Rob told him. "The other trucks decided to drive right in front of us just now, and made a new track!"

We enjoyed a high-spirited exchange before the huge vehicle charged its engine and rumbled away.

Rob walked along slowly, still waving to the driver, but I glanced backwards and got the shock of my life. The huge rear wheel of the tanker had nudged up beside the old Toyota and rolled forward, folding the front and rear passenger doors of our little truck back against its body and crumpling the whole side in. At any moment the old vehicle could topple on its side!

"Stop! Stop!" I howled, my voice drowning in the sound of the engines. "*STOP!*"

Rob was startled as I ran by, until he too looked back and realized what was happening. Finally I caught the attention of the driver in his side mirror. The big truck ground to a halt and the driver looked out.

"Your wheel damaged our vehicle," I told him, pointing. "Look!"

He got out of his rig and his gaze followed my trembling finger.

"Sorry! Sorry!" he repeated, and then, suddenly, the import of his actions dawned on him. His tone changed.

"But those aren't my tracks!" he protested.

Funny, you seem to be the only one here, I thought. By this time Rob had caught up and I passed the conversation over to him while I dived for a camera to capture the evidence.

"I will have to get a police report," he said to the truck driver. "Where is the nearest police station?"

It was imperative to have this paper, for without it the Toyota could be impounded by police if they noticed it was damaged. We could be in serious trouble if we didn't have proof of what had caused the accident. The driver, resigning himself to the strength of the evidence against him, begged us not to go to the police.

"I will get a fine and maybe I will lose my job," he protested. "I will pay for the repair myself."

"But that doesn't help me when I go back through a town," Rob said. "What if the police see me and start asking questions? Call your supervisor on the radio and we'll talk to him."

The morning was half gone by the time the matter was settled. The driver would pay for all damages but we still needed a police report, which we could get from a tiny police station up the road, in the middle of nowhere.

The rear door could be tied in place but the inside handles of the front passenger and driver's doors had to be tied together, across our laps, to keep them closed. Even then sand blew in. It was an uncomfortable drive down to *Shaybah* but we decided to carry on and see the new compound anyway.

As we traveled south, the wind began to paint striking patterns with coarse red and dense white sand between the dunes, which increased in size until they became sand mountains. They rose to over six hundred feet high, and between them lay *subkha*, potentially boggy ground.

The construction company building the road to *Shaybah* was gradually working its way north from the oilfield and we passed their camp on the way down. When we hit the completed stretch of road we sped along and were soon peering down on a valley containing a flurry of construction and rows of temporary buildings.

We drove cautiously up to what might be the administration building and knocked on the door.

An American supervisor received us graciously into his air-conditioned aluminum cocoon and happily discussed the development of the project over cold refreshments. The *Shaybah* oilfield is one of the largest in the world, with reserves of more than fourteen billion barrels of crude oil and twenty-five trillion cubic feet of gas. The crude is Arabian extra light, high-quality grade oil.

Considering that the site of the compound was five hundred miles from *Dhahran*, the construction project was phenomenal. On completion it would have housing facilities for over seven hundred employees, administrative offices, an air-strip, a fire station, recreation areas, maintenance and support shops, and stations for power generation and distribution. There would also be a four hundred mile fiber-optic cable linking *Shaybah* to the main radio system at *Abqaiq* in the north.

The supervisor also told us that the growing community consumed a huge amount of water per day and that this had to be trucked in because the groundwater was contaminated with radiation. This requirement would doubtless provide the trucking company with secure, long-term employment.

There was little reason to remain after our meeting, so we decided to head north again.

"Let's stop and say hello to the guys at the construction site," Rob suggested.

The road construction was under a European contractor, who was happy to speak with us.

"What happened to your truck?" he asked. When Rob explained, he shook his head.

"Let one of my guys work on it for you," he said. "They have all the equipment they need to straighten out your doors, at least so you can close them without tying them up. And while you are waiting, go over and eat at the canteen. There is plenty of food."

We thanked him for his kindness and enjoyed a hot meal in the mobile cafeteria. Then our new friend found us again.

"There is a sand storm coming," he said. "Why don't you stay with us for the night? It's going to be very windy and you may not be able to find your way out tonight. We have spare cabins here. Tomorrow you can follow the convoy out."

We accepted his hospitality, overwhelmed by his generosity and the fact that he would not let us pay for anything. Rob happened to have a flask of his quality *siddiqi*, homemade alcohol, hidden away in a lunchbox.

"Would you like this?" he asked.

"It's a long time since I could drink alcohol!" he said, eyes wide.

"You will need to dilute it, it is full strength," Rob warned as the supervisor disappeared with the bottle, a smile on his face. We wondered how much he had understood of our English instructions.

It was very comfortable in the cabins. I lay quietly, grateful for the protection from the blasting sand, and listened to the wind howling outside. When

I awakened, the skies were clear again and the convoy was marking a new trail amongst the dunes.

As we left the camp and headed out in our modified vehicle, the supervisor wandered in to work. He had bleary eyes, tousled hair and a very obvious hangover. He had clearly not followed Bob's instructions exactly, on diluting the *sid*. But he was a very happy man.

44 - A HOLE IN ONE

IT WAS MAY and already very hot. It was too late to go camping but we wanted to survey the Mossy Dahl, which we had discovered two years previously.

"The temperature will be cooler below ground than above," Rob said. "No different from the temperature in winter. We can spend the hottest part of the days in the *dahl*."

It was odd going by ourselves. Usually we entered the desert with at least one other vehicle, and a shiver of apprehension ran over me as we set off. All was quiet as we set up camp the first night; even the owls had found cooler digs for the summer. A campfire seemed foolish but we lit one anyway, to cook and to boil water for tea.

As we lay on our old army cots in the open air the stars blazed bright under the velvety-black canopy of the heavens. I spent no more than a moment thinking of camel spiders before I fell asleep.

The sun woke me up early, more by its heat than its light. Rob was halfway to the dunes before I swung my legs over the side of my cot and yawned.

My shoes were upside down and I shook them out. A scorpion fell out of one of them, recovered itself, and ambled off to find a less turbulent residence for the day.

The sand was already shimmering by the time we'd eaten breakfast and made our way to the entrance of the *dahl*. The temperature contrast was not enough now to create any moisture at the entrance and winter's bright green mossy ring had gone dry and black.

It was cooler inside the cave but still warm enough to make us sweat in our helmets and long sleeves. We tried out 'the loudest whistle in the world,' which we'd bought in Canada, and discovered the sound would not penetrate through rock. I switched off my headlight and the blackness was so dense I could feel it.

And then we began surveying using a compass, a long tape measure, and a level with a tiny laser light strapped to it. Like rabbits in a warren we squirmed along narrow passages in a pall of silence broken only by the sounds of breathing and an occasional exchange of conversation.

After a picnic lunch we fell asleep for a while on the floor of the cave before continuing our work. The cave system was surprisingly small and we wondered just how many other insignificant holes in the ground were hiding similar caves. When we finally emerged the sun was low in the sky and the temperature was tolerable.

Next morning we headed north and after an hour or so of bumping along a desert track we noticed a long, dark Bedouin tent. Three women at its entrance were startled by our appearance. Rob got out of the vehicle and walked slowly toward them, calling out in Arabic.

One of the women, an old lady, stood her ground while the two younger women retreated to the safety of the tent. We discovered that the man of the establishment was away but would be back soon and we were welcome to sit and wait for him in the tent and have a cup or three of coffee.

We stayed and engaged the old lady in conversation. She was delightfully blunt. After giving us a brief history of her family she informed us that her three daughters were as yet unmarried.

"They are waiting for Americans," she said, guffawing with laughter.

When we told her that we were exploring caves she became alarmed.

"Don't go in there!" she exclaimed. "You will die!"

When the man of the house arrived he readily agreed to show Rob where more *dahls* were.

"You two go in the Land Cruiser," I said. "You can get GPS positions on the caves and I will wait here and talk with the ladies while you're gone."

It was an hour or more before they returned. The two younger women came out into the sitting area of the tent and we sought windows into each others' worlds in Arabic. More tea and coffee appeared; more dates and goats' cheese.

"How old are your daughters?" I asked the old lady.

"One is twenty two, the other is twenty-four," she said. "They want to get married but the dowry is high and men have to save up a long time to afford a wife in these parts."

It was a hard life in the desert, and I guessed that in time the young Bedou would gradually drift to the cities where life was easier and not as lonely.

Rob and his host returned with two more interesting holes pinpointed on the GPS and we set off to explore them, to the consternation of the old lady.

"Please, don't go inside those holes!" she entreated again.

One turned out to be a blind pit, and when Rob belayed me down the second I discovered the bottom to be full of stagnant water. There also seemed to be a horizontal shaft leading away from me but my flashlight was not strong enough to illuminate it and I had no way of reaching it. The best I could do was to snap a photograph and hope that something showed up on film. (It turned out to have a blind end.)

A low rocky shelf jutted out from the wall a little further down and, as there was nothing else to see below it and the wet bottom of the *dahl*, I swung myself over onto it. Since completing my rappelling course I had not had the opportunity to try my ascender and now I threaded it onto my ropes with trembling hands. It took longer than I expected. Rob called down the shaft anxiously.

"It's OK," I yelled. "I just have to figure this thing out."

When I thought I had it correctly assembled I tested my weight on it and crept upwards a few inches. Whew—it worked!

"I'm ready!" I called. "I'm coming up."

I began the caterpillar crawl up the long rope but towards the top of the *dahl* the shaft narrowed so my arms were pinned down. My legs started to shake uncontrollably.

"I can haul you the rest of the way," Rob said. "You aren't very heavy."

I finally fell out of the vertical shaft and collapsed onto level ground, panting.

"No *Jinn* down there?" he joked as he helped me out of my harness.

We stopped at the Bedouin tent briefly, to reassure the Bedou that we were indeed still alive after our perilous descent into the *dahls*, and began the six-hour journey back to Ras Tanura.

45 - EXIT ONLY

ROB WAS SITTING in his armchair after work, looking as smug as the cat after a good meal. He held out a letter for me to read. I stared at it blankly for a moment. Then the significance of it struck me like a bullet.

"You did it!" I exclaimed. "You made the surplus list!"

"We've got until the end of December," he said, no longer holding back the grin. "Plenty of time to work through the Exit Only list."

I couldn't believe it. A mixture of emotions swirled around me. Now we would be able to take up residency in our islands in the sun!

But it would be a monumental upheaval in our lives. We would never be able to return—we would have to leave our car, home, neighbors and friends as we cut the umbilical cord to "Mother Aramco." For so long all of our needs had been supplied in housing, maintenance, medical, vacations, shipping, recreation and livelihood.

The experience of others had taught us how traumatic this separation could be. And part of me hated the thought of leaving this country which had become my home. We were about to be tossed into the big, wide world.

There were three months to sort and pack and it fell on me to do the inventory, as Rob still had to go to work. This meant long days of itemizing everything in the house, listing each with a value, country of origin and where it was to be shipped to. Everything we owned down to the last pair of socks had to be listed for the company's shipping records.

Rob had been with the company for over eighteen years and had been collecting things ever since he'd arrived in Kingdom. I had no idea what some of his treasures were or where they had come from and frequently had to call him at work to ask. The lists grew and grew.

We left the grand piano with Canadian friends.

"We'll bring it back to Canada with our shipment when we leave," they promised. "You can collect it when you come to live in Canada."

Days and weeks went by in a blur. Finally we submitted the inventory forms and settled on a packing date. Then Ramadan approached and the work wheel slowed almost to a halt. The time arrived to hand in our ID cards and get temporary papers. Rob took them to Personnel while I was busy with other things.

"Your wife has to come here too and sign," said the young man at the counter.

"I'll go and get her now," Rob sighed, and returned with me a few minutes later.

"We are leaving now," said the Personnel officer. "We finish at one o'clock during Ramadan. You'll have to come back tomorrow."

The next day we showed up early in the morning, to be greeted with a puzzled stare from another employee.

"You don't need your wife here. It's OK—we just need your ID cards."

Around this time I also had to make a decision—what to do with Hobie. He was now almost two years old and a fine looking animal but just as timid as he had been as a kitten. I tried hard to find a home for him and yet I feared that he would run away as he had from Gary. If he ran from a new home after we had left Kingdom there would be nowhere for him to go and he would either starve to death or become so weak that wild dogs could finish him off.

I couldn't bear the thought. I called around and discovered that many employees were leaving, and that finding homes for even pedigreed animals was proving difficult. There was only one thing to do. Hobie had to be put to sleep.

"No!" cried a friend. "There's an excellent animal psychologist in New York—take him there! I'm sure he could be treated for his shyness."

But a trip to America for a cat psychologist was out of the question. I got some sedatives from the vet as I had done when Hobie had been neutered. Double the dose this time, to be given an hour and a half before the vet appointment. The vet also gave me a syringe with another sedative to inject under the skin. I had never given an injection before.

"Pull up the skin around his neck and jab the needle in quickly. He won't even feel it," said the vet. "And do it around the same time as you give him the tablets."

The afternoon arrived and I prepared the deadly medication. I put the syringe behind me on the floor so that Hobie would not become nervous, and gathered him into my arms. He purred softly, gazing up at me with slightly crossed blue eyes, and I felt my heart breaking. *Perfect trust.* Trust which I was about to betray.

I pried open his jaws gently and stuffed the tablets down his throat. He made a small sound and stiffened a little, then swallowed uneasily as he took up his position on my lap again. *Now.* Taking the syringe with a trembling hand, I gathered up the skin around his neck as I'd been told to.

Rrrrinnggg! Who *was* that person at the front door? Hobie's body contracted into a ball of muscle and he would have catapulted from my arms and out into the garden if I had not held onto him with all my might. He had never once extended his claws against me and he did not do it now.

"Rob!" I yelled frantically, "Get the door! Send them away!"

Rob stirred slowly in the office upstairs and the bell rang again.

"Hurry!" I cried. "Right now—*please!*" Hobie struggled more frantically. *That's all I need. The cat will escape and go to sleep who-knows-where and the whole plan will fall apart.*

Rob finally went outside with his guest and all was quiet. Hobie began to relax and my heart slowed. My hand was shaking so badly the first time I drove the syringe downward that the needle only grazed the skin. Hobie gave a puzzled growl and stiffened again.

"It's OK, Hobie," I said, stroking him back into position. My second attempt was successful. I heaved a sigh of relief as the last of the liquid left the syringe.

"My poor boy," I whispered, tears streaming from my eyes.

Upstairs in the bathroom I turned on the night light and there caressed Hobie until his body loosened. As he began to lose control of his limbs I wrapped him in a towel and left him to rest.

Rob had to take Hobie into the vet's office. I could not see for crying and waited in the car.

"He was so zonked out I am sure he had no idea what was going on," said Rob when he came back alone. "The vet gave him extra dope to make sure he had really succumbed. There's no doubt about it now, you can be sure he's finished."

Although it was the best thing for everyone under the circumstances, including Hobie, I still feel a twinge of sadness at the thought of the beautiful, gentle animal whose life was all too short.

But duty called and there were other things to occupy our minds. There were farewell dinners and presentations, goodbye speeches and gifts. Leaving Aramco began to feel like a slow form of amputation and I grieved for the separation which had already begun to tear us apart. Smiling faces before me blurred through my tears.

And then it was time for the garage sale. I hated it. People picked over our stuff, offering less and less for things that were already under-priced, knowing that we were leaving and had to sell.

"Too much! Too much!" crowed a man who came to look at the microwave.

"Don't buy it then," I said.

I could see he wanted it badly but was unwilling to pay a fair price for it. He hesitated a long time before passing over the money.

A woman whined about a handful of items until I practically gave them to her and another came in and offered a pittance for whatever was left in the room.

These people were, I discovered, old hands at garage sales, and bought and resold regularly. Even Suwara, the woman who placed the notices on the board in the mail centre, would try to buy things for almost nothing before she placed the notices then send the goods home to Sudan for resale there.

When I couldn't take any more of the aggravation, I gave the rest to our charity group to use in their next garage sale. Better to donate to charity and preserve one's sanity than to allow the vultures free reign. I can imagine how it feels for those in bankruptcy to watch their possessions sold at fire-sale prices.

It seemed like an endless game of snakes and ladders, with more snakes than ladders. A new rule forbade expatriates to leave the country exit-only while still owning a car. There must be proof of sale as too many rusting hulks had been dumped at the airport, never to be reclaimed, as the owners had left for good.

One thing that particularly saddened us was the loss of our planned trip to Oman the month after our departure.

"It would be good if we could defer our exit-only visa somehow," said Rob thoughtfully. "We could leave Saudi Arabia, do the Oman trip then come back, sell the car and leave."

He called several friends in high places but was referred on to others who might be able to help. Finally he gave up and made our departure the conventional way—booking flights out of Dhahran for our last day of employment with the company. And finally our old Toyota was sold.

And then the packers came—a team of Pakistanis who swept into the house like a tornado, wrapping and boxing our goods. The boxes began to stack up in the van outside and the house gradually emptied.

I had very little contact with my friends in Dhahran during those last days. Every night I fell into bed late and exhausted, and the days melted into each other.

We checked off items on our "to do" list. Exit medical examinations, return library cards, Personnel checks, Security checks, Government affairs, close bank accounts, garage sale, repaint, inventory, packing, housing inspections and clearance, airline bookings...there was more to do than seemed possible but finally the last morning dawned.

The last snag we struck was a miscommunication between two computers regarding our car sale, two days before we were due to leave. Rob had spent two days rushing about, trying to convince Aramco that the car had been sold and that the proof of sale was on the computer in Rahima, even if it didn't show in Dammam. Finally he burst into the house, only an hour before we were scheduled to leave for the airport.

"Here are our exit-only visas!" he called triumphantly, waving a signed form in the air.

I'd used every last minute packing, cleaning, delivering left-over items and saying goodbye to friends who'd called in. We were isolated now, with no telephone. There were few neighbors left on our street and I remembered with a pang that Maria had asked me to call on our way out of the country.

But the taxi arrived before I could make an excursion down to the telephone at the mail centre. We piled our luggage into the vehicle, squeezed ourselves in after it, and sped through the gates of Ras Tanura before I had time to reflect. Casting a regretful glance back at the place which was so full of memories for me, I wondered if the shock of leaving would equal the shock of arriving in the first place.

After picking up our passports in Dhahran, we headed for the causeway across the Arabian Gulf to Bahrain. The desert was soon behind us and we could finally relax as the highway flew by. It was almost an anticlimax when we walked into the airport. Just another plane trip, I thought. It could have been any repat or short leave.

We settled into our seats on the aircraft, and I leaned back and closed my eyes. Once again I was back on the dunes in the Rub Al Khali, listening to the wind moan as it lifted sand particles into the air, sifting and transporting them relentlessly onward.

Part of me belonged here, would always belong here. And then the whirr of the wind became the drone of the engines and a fierce stab shot through my chest. It was time to leave this troubled and beautiful country which had somehow become my own.

"We are all strange or we wouldn't be here," Rob had often said, and now we were not to be here any longer. That felt very strange indeed.

END